Death on a Fork

And how to avoid it!

Death on a Fork

And how to avoid it!

Gwynne H. Davies DSc ND DO
Clinical Ecologist – Retired

BOOKS

Winchester, UK
Washington, USA

First published by O-Books, 2011
O-Books is an imprint of John Hunt Publishing Ltd., Laurel House, Station Approach,
Alresford, Hants, SO24 9JH, UK
office1@o-books.net
www.o-books.com

For distributor details and how to order please visit the 'Ordering' section on our website.

ISBN: 978 1 84694 837 4

A CIP catalogue record for this book is available from the British Library.

Design: Stuart Davies

Printed in the UK by CPI Antony Rowe
Printed in the USA by Offset Paperback Mfrs, Inc

CONTENTS

Acknowledgements

Many of you will be aware that my last book, *Allergies – Breakthrough to Health,* was published in 2004. This was after much soul searching, and now six years later it is more apparent than ever that it needs rewriting and updating a great deal.

My dear wife Rosemarie has "encouraged" me to do this for some time now as have Jenny and Tony, and Sean and Kazy, thank you for your input and inspiration. I also have to thank Dr Andrew Tresidder and Dr Michael Stewardson for their contributions in writing the forewords.

It is hard to believe but I am in my 81st year now so I have had some time to explore and hopefully have learnt that advances have been made and I must move with the times. It has also given me time to bring myself up to date on what is going on in this world of ours. One thing that is very clear to me is that allergies, or if you prefer, food sensitivity, is more prevalent since I retired. Obesity seems to be the "In" word, according to the press almost epidemic. Take my word for it this does not need to be the case and there are several very good reasons for it.

To use a phrase I use consistently throughout this book and my three others – YOU DO NOT HAVE TO LIVE WITH IT!! If you are willing to take the bull by the horns and adjust the way that you eat then you have every chance to change your health and life style.

There are many unsolicited letters herein and to those and all my patients in the past and present – thank you for your support and patience. I have read many books and find them most confusing and as yet have not read one that is based on 30 years of practical hands on treatment. This book is not hypothesis it is factual based on the correlation of facts deduced from my patients over that period and since I retired.

VIZ MEDICATRIX NATURAE

The healing power of nature – Hippocrates.

Foreword

Food allergy and intolerance is a massively important subject that can affect every one of us.

Now that that we all realise that we all have a responsibility for our own health, it is vital to learn simple ways that can help us. Most of us take our health for granted until there is a problem – and it is human nature to ask someone else to help sort it out.

Modern medicine and surgery have produced wonders – but until now we have been so busy with the technological angles that society has undervalued, or even ignored, basic issues such as how foods can affect us.

Medicine has followed Pasteur in blaming "the germ" as the cause of illness. After all when something goes wrong, it's nice to find someone else to blame! However on his deathbed Pasteur said "Bernard was right – it is not just the seed, but the soil that is important". By this he meant that Claude Bernard was right in emphasising the importance of the general health of the body. If you're really healthy, it is more difficult for bacteria or viruses to take hold.

We all need to remember that "we are what we eat "and that the body has its own tremendous ability to heal itself – the "Vis Medicatrix Naturae".

I took my health for granted, until aged thirty; mumps laid me low for three months. Mumps as an adult is not fun! After recovering, I developed headaches on a daily basis. By chance, I read Dr Richard Mackarness' book "Not all in the Mind", all about food intolerances. Also by chance, a friend used Gwynne Davies' test on me. I was amazed to find that my body could lose strength as a reaction to certain foods. I was even more amazed that giving up those foods cured my headaches.

Gwynne Davies has done us all a great service, by painstaking observation, by development of a system of diagnosis and cure, and by helping thousands of people. Even better, he has chosen to share his findings with us, to help more of us to understand how we can be helped – and how we can help ourselves.

Firm foundations are essential to any building. Likewise, healthy nutrition tailored to the individual is essential to maintain health. Indeed, as Gwynne has found, sometimes right nutrition (eliminating food intolerances) is the only thing that may be needed to make us substantially better. By eliminating a daily negative, the body's power of self healing is free to accentuate the positive.

Increasingly people ask doctors how they can help themselves. Discovering and doing something about our food intolerances is a very positive thing we can do ourselves. Learning about nutrition is going to be a growth area for the rest of the century – and science is starting to be interested.

By picking up this book you've already shown yourself that you're ahead of the game! Good luck to you, and good health! And thank you Gwynne for writing this book!

Dr Andrew Tresidder. Chard 2002.

Author's comment.

Thank you Andrew for those kind comments. 2002 seems a long way away now, and with those passing years I wish I could report that nutrition was being accepted far more by the medical establishment, sadly this does not appear to be the case. What worries me is that all the press reports I read state that allergies/food sensitivity are getting worse. Obesity is pandemic. Chlamydia is rife. Campylobacter is still prevalent. Cancer is escalating. Surely it is not beyond the realms that the media take it upon themselves to announce that all of these conditions are treatable, and in many cases resolved by the individual taking responsibility for their health.

You mentioned Claude Bernard and the soil being so

important. If the Ph of the soil is not correct then the plant (health) cannot grow.

We create our future body by what we eat.

We become what we do not excrete.

This makes the poem below very apposite.

AN ANCIENT PRAYER
Give me a good digestion Lord
And also something to digest
Give me a healthy body Lord
With sense to keep it at its best
Give me a healthy mind Lord
To keep the good and pure in sight
Which seeing wrong is not appalled?
But finds a way to put it right
Give me a mind that is not bored
That does not whimper, whine or sigh
Don't let me worry over much
About the fussy thing called "I"
Give me a sense of humour Lord
Give me the grace to see a joke
To get some happiness out of life
And pass it on to other folk
Anonymous

Chapter 1

What is a Clinical Ecologist?

A Clinical Ecologist is a holistic consultant who aims to restore perfect balance to the physical, emotional and spiritual aspects of the human being. Thereby treating any disease or illness of the human condition and aiming to achieve the best quality of life for as long as possible.

Which brings me to the attitudes expressed by certain sections of the media? In a tabloid newspaper on Tuesday February 9th, 2010 the headlines shrieked THE GREAT FOOD ALLERGY MYTH by Matthew Barbour. This article intimated throughout that allergy/food sensitivity was all in the mind. That comment alone takes me back to the foreword by Dr Andrew Tresidder referring to the book by Dr Richard Mackarness – Not All in the Mind. For those of you who read this book you will remember that after intensive research at Park Prewett Hospital it certainly was not all in the mind.

If this were to be the case I wonder why very few weeks go by that we are not reminded on radio and television that the allergy/food sensitivity problem is getting worse, and, referred to on one programme as being pandemic. The article I referred to in the previous paragraph did have the grace to admit that the doctors referred to did not know the answers either, and all their comments were based on supposition.

Forgive me if I am repeating myself but in this book you will not find supposition – you will find the clinical evidence I accrued over a thirty year period, no hypothesis, actual testing results. Some of the points mentioned in the article are valid. Because you are reacting to a particular food it does not necessarily mean you have to eliminate the whole group of related foods. This is where individual assessment and testing are so valuable. Having said that, my advice in the early stages of elimination was to avoid the relevant group in toto, then when the symptoms had totally disappeared – slowly – introduces them one at a time making sure there is no tangible reaction. Not, and I repeat not the suspect food itself.

We know it isn't, but if it were all a myth why was I kept so busy seeing on average ten to twelve patients daily and had a waiting list of four months when I retired? I would suggest that perhaps my methodology does not fit any recognised and scientifically proven method, but my contention is that success is measured by whether you get the patient well or not, and we certainly did that most of the time. The major part of the article that attracted my attention was the statements by one doctor that far too many people were being told they were sensitive to dairy products, milk in particular, and this was wrong. Dr Judith Bryans of the Dairy Council made the following statement "adolescence is a critical period for laying the foundation for future bone health, as at least 90% of bone mass in girls is achieved by 18 years of age. Milk and dairy foods are some of the best dietary sources of bone-building nutrients such as calcium, phosphorous and protein". Being cynical but truthful, she would say that wouldn't she being on the Dairy Council.

I would ask her to compare the calcium, phosphorous and protein levels in sheep or goat milk. The difference is so minute it is not worth considering. I am a member and contributor to The Physicians Committee for Responsible Medicine in the USA, and they, along with other medical periodicals in the UK have been saying for years that the evidence points to milk and dairy products as being deleterious to health. Headline in the UK press – "Doctors Link Cow's Milk to Diabetes". Research from the University of Rome and St Bartholomew's Hospital in London published in the Lancet provides a scientific explanation of why this could happen. "According to new research people with diabetes do have immune cells that seem primed to attack a cow's milk protein called beta casein, which resembles the pancreatic beta cell protein". What is one of the most prevalent diseases today? – Diabetes.

My hypothesis has always been that the genetic IgE factor along with IgA was responsible for producing a pancreatic malfunction and hence a breakdown in the immune system. The whole of my practice life and approach to symptomology was to address the possibility of a pancreatic malfunction. How right I was. Nothing has changed even though I have been retired for fifteen years all the evidence points to dairy as a major culprit – more later. Suffice to say I will never be made a Freeman of the Dairy Council.

Understanding disease

The chronic effects of stress, pollution, faulty diet or unhappiness are subtle and do not begin to make themselves felt until the chain breaks at its weakest link, and pathology shows itself in one form or another. To look at the pathology in isolation is to examine only a slice of what is in fact a continuum of events, and it is important to realise that the same stimulus has been affecting other aspects of the body which may only fail later. I guarantee that when a patient presents with a condition such as rheumatoid arthritis that would be the only condition they would be worried about. But, on detailed questioning going back over years it was almost always the case that minor and subtle symptoms had been evident and that the breakdown of the immune system had begun a long time ago. It was not until that crucial "straw that broke the camel's back" occurred that the pain and discomfort were enough to require a consultation.

Therefore to try and reverse that particular symptom without looking beyond is of limited value, although it may be worth addressing the rheumatoid arthritis as such, it only gains in real value if we spend more time looking at the events that led to the breakdown , background history is so important. You will hear me mention this statement many times throughout this book but it is a truism that as far as I am concerned is indisputable – **Find the Cause!**

What is Allergy?

The word allergy is often used loosely, people are said to be allergic to anything that does not agree with them. From this has grown the metaphorical or jokey sense in which we speak of a lazy person being "allergic" to hard work, or the mother in law. The true meaning of allergy is more precise; it is the condition in which a person's immune system regards an ordinary harmless substance as a dangerous "invader" and responds to it by producing antibodies, which in their turn give rise to unpleasant reactions.

The most severe is anaphylactic shock an extreme and generalised allergic reaction in which widespread histamine release causes swelling (oedema), constriction of the bronchioles, heart failure, circulatory collapse and sometimes death. Thankfully this reaction is rare but can be brought about by a bee or wasp sting. In each case help should be sought IMMEDIATELY! Ring 999 – send an ambulance – suspect anaphylactic reaction – send ambulance or paramedic immediately. It is possible that the person affected is aware of this reaction and carries an Epipen which is adrenaline and contained in an oblong yellow box. Read the instruction leaflet and inject in to patients buttock, rub the injection site vigorously to disperse the adrenaline. It is a safety injection, so do not be afraid, in all probability you will save a life, and do no harm. But – **speed is of the essence!**

Asthma, Eczema and hay fever are perhaps the best known manifestations of an allergic reaction. But in fact the full range of reactions is much more devious and complicated. Immunologists work mainly on the basis that extraneous elements such as animal dander, house dust mite, pollens etc; cause an allergic response. I hope to show in this book that while many people are affected by these substances, their reactions are often caused by an underlying food sensitivity "trigger" which provides the breeding ground for these extraneous reactions.

Let me give you a classic example. Soon after I met my wife Rosemarie we were invited to a friend's house for the evening. They had cats for many years but knowing Rosemarie had been an asthmatic since early childhood they made sure the cats were out of the house for hours before we arrived. We had not been in the house for more than half an hour when it became apparent that a reaction was occurring. Her nose started to run, her eyes were watering and she started to wheeze and needing to use an inhaler. A classic reaction.

Once we had found out the basic "triggers" and many months later she was stable in that type of situation and we have owned two cats ever since. Or should I say they have owned us.

I would like to explain in as uncomplicated way as possible the General Adaptation Syndrome, commonly called the Stress Syndrome. This is described fully by Professor Hans Selye of Montreal University and adapted and used by Theron Randolph (known as the father of clinical ecology) as the Specific Adaptation Syndrome in his book Human Ecology and Susceptibility to the Chemical Environment. Both of these are large tomes so I will try and simplify it as much as possible.

There are three stages.

Stage I
Alarm Reaction

This could be experienced in a number of ways but the one that most people recognise is a reaction to strawberries manifesting as a rash or swollen mouth. One of the most typical and to my mind the most overlooked, is the baby that projectile vomits after feeding. The mother assumes it is just an upset stomach and continues to feed the baby cow's milk and cow's milk products.

After some time the projectile vomiting ceases and it is naturally assumed the child has "grown out of it". Then either a nappy rash or eczema appears. The child has moved on to the next stage.

Stage 2
Adaptation

This is the stage of adaptation where although toxins (poisons) are being ingested the body only shows minor reactions. The adrenal glands situated on top of the kidneys are able to cope by producing enough adrenaline, cortisone and histamine to keep the system functioning and reasonably stable. Over the days, weeks and months, depending on the amount of toxins being ingested, the adrenal glands slowly atrophy (shrink) to the size of a hazelnut instead of a healthy walnut, then inevitably we drop in to the next stage.

Stage 3
Exhaustion

At the same time the mast cells that we have compartmentalised throughout the body are being attacked by the antibodies that are being produced. These antibodies slowly but surely coat the mast cells until two extremely important things occur. The adrenal glands have atrophied and the mast cells become fully coated – an explosion occurs – the mast cells shrug off the antibodies and they flood in to the system.

By the mast cells being compartmentalised the following simple explanation may help. Mast cells in the head – migraine, headaches, neurological conditions. Chest – bronchitis, asthma. Gut – irritable bowel syndrome, Crohns disease, constipation, diarrhoea. A generalised reaction would probably produce arthritis/ rheumatoid or hyperactivity, short attention span, physical aggression.

It is my hypothesis that it is in a Stage 1 reaction that a

pancreatic malfunction occurs and "triggers" the whole process. It is in these compromised reactions that the immune system is unable to respond correctly and the stroking of a cat or dog would indeed precipitate a reaction.

A young lad I shall call John, came to see me with an asthmatic condition which had been apparent since early childhood. It was exacerbated by proximity to cats, dogs and horses. The last was the one that annoyed him the most was because he had a real connection with horses and from childhood wanted to become a jockey. But, it did not bode well if he went near a horse. His nose would stream like a tap, his eyes would water and itch and he would wheeze. I explained to John and his parents about the "trigger" factor and proceeded to test John. He was allergic/sensitive to all dairy products. In those days white flour contained 52 additives and preservatives and he was allergic to that too. I am delighted to say that since those days these have been removed. After three weeks of eliminating these toxins in total he was not only able to go near a horse but joy of joys, he could actually ride one without any reaction. He has since become a successful jockey.

I am not suggesting that all conditions are allergy related, neither that all reactions are food sensitivity related. But the majority of chronic conditions have an underlying causatory "trigger". This why it was so important to take a careful case history and note all pre-disposing symptoms. They invariably tell a sorry tale of long term suffering that thankfully can be ameliorated. In my 30 years in practice I never wavered from that premise, testing thousands of patients and achieving results almost immediately. Bearing in mind of course, that 90% of patients had been there and had the t-shirt, having gone through all the "normal" procedures with no resolution – x-rays, barium meal, blood tests, enema, MRI Scan etc; in other words at the end of their tether. But on carrying out the pancreatic malfunction test the path was immediately open to recovery. I regularly saw

10-12 patients daily and carried a waiting list of three to four months and I felt that this indicated some marked degree of success.

WHAT ARE THE MOST COMMON ALLERGY REACTIONS?

Nasal catarrh & Hay Fever

There are many hundreds of people who only suffer with this complaint when the pollen count is high. Roughly from May to September - the "hay fever season". The symptoms differ from the common cold in that the mucous tends to be thin and watery, the eyes become red and irritable, and sneezing bouts are frequent and at times lengthy. Modern anti-histamine drugs usually take care of the worst symptoms and thankfully these days do not cause drowsiness or affect the concentration level. Is this really the answer? No of course it isn't, no drug is acceptable as a panacea, and all drugs have inherent side effects. So the answer is "find the cause" and eliminate it. In the back of the book you will find a list of clinical ecologists trained by me who will be able to find that elusive "trigger" for you. One word of caution. It is very rare for a patient to recover and strengthen the immune system enough unless they have carried out a detoxification programme for at least three months beforehand.

Asthma and Bronchial Congestion

This is a distressing condition which causes sufferers a deal of alarm. I find it difficult to imagine what it must be like not being able to breathe properly, panic, apprehension, unless one has suffered with this condition it is hard to imagine. They wheeze and have a sensation of a tight band around the chest and throat. This is due to inflammation of the bronchi producing a muscular spasm, an effect that can be likened cramp in the leg or other parts of the body. The frequent attacks are often associated with stress, or excitement, in some cases induced by laughter. This gives the impression that external stress is the cause. I am sure that there are occasions when this is true, conversely I would suggest that if the causatory "trigger" was removed, and the adrenal glands and mast cells are not dropping in to Stage 3 (exhaustion), the patients need for inhalers is reduced, and in some cases eliminated, the general health of the patient improves considerably.

Eczema, dermatitis, psoriasis

In this painful and unsightly group of ailments the skin is subject to extreme irritation. Scratching can cause bleeding and inflammation which frequently leads to infection. In the majority of cases it has manifested since early childhood. I wish I had a pound for every patient I have heard say, "I was told I would grow out of it" or "Use a cream or emollient and it will reduce the irritation and eventually go away". Apart from anything else it becomes extremely difficult to protect bedding or clothing. In many cases the ointment is a corticosteroid or steroid based cream that has the deleterious effect of thinning the skin, and being absorbed through the derma to produce internal problems.

In my experience it is totally wrong to suggest that one grows out of anything. Whether it is after seven, fourteen or twenty one years. What actually happens is that one particular set of mast cells comes under attack and becomes saturated and the antibodies move on to another set of mast cells. How many times have I heard from patients "I had eczema as a child but I grew out of it"? My next question is always to ask what they are suffering from now and why they need to see me. Inevitably it has moved to a more serious condition like asthma or arthritis or an internal problem. It has "moved house".

The worst case of eczema I ever saw was a Professor from Manchester University. He was literally covered from head to foot, suppurating and necessitating using bandages around his ankles to mop up. Needless to say the smell was quite unpleasant and an acute embarrassment to the poor man. He was on heavy ointment use and medication, all of which were lactose based. He was lactose intolerant and they were worsening the condition. Because of inactivity he had put on an enormous amount of weight and his liver was malfunctioning. In fact he was in a bad way. Needless to say he was so relieved to find the underlying causatory "triggers". Above all for him to appreciate that we had found the cause and he was going to get better. He came back six weeks later having lost one and a half stone and apart from odd patches on the arms and legs he was clear. He continued to lose weight and the eczema cleared completely over a period of six months.

A point that is very difficult for such patients to appreciate is, that the derma is the first indication that the immune system is under attack. So, by addressing that situation they are preventing more serious complications. It is there early warning system.

Spastic colon, Ulcerative colitis, bloating, irritable bowel syndrome, Crohns disease.

Symptoms can be intermittent diarrhoea and constipation, soreness of the anus with a discharge (pruritus), pains in the lower abdomen which can be spasmodic and extremely painful. (Gut migraine). Also food going through the system undigested, bloating even after a light meal, a feeling of having a lump in the throat (frequently diagnosed as hiatus hernia). In severe cases such as Crohns disease there is often blood and mucus in the faeces. Whilst this latter condition is the most severe, it is nearly always the easiest condition to resolve, and in a comparatively short space of time. I am reminded of a teacher who had continual diarrhoea which was extremely weakening and left her worn out, urticaria (hives) and nausea all the time. I found she was sensitive to many foods but the major culprit was wheat, and after eliminating these foods the "triggers" she is now symptom free and able to resume her teaching career. After the onset of this nasty condition she had been prescribed three courses of antibiotics and sadly these had not resolved the problem.

I would go as far as to say that in my experience antibiotics rarely cure a gut condition, and in many cases actually exacerbate it.

I would like to give you the dictionary description of Crohns disease: - "a condition in which segments of the alimentary tract become inflamed thickened and ulcerated. It usually affects the terminal part of the ileum; its acute form (acute ileitis) may mimic appendicitis. Chronic disease often causes partial obstruction of the intestine, leading to pain, diarrhoea and malabsorption. Fistulae around the anus, between adjacent loops of intestine, or from intestine to skin, bladder etc; are characteristic complications. The cause is unknown. Treatment includes rest, corticosteroids, immunosuppressive drugs, antibiotics, dietary modification, or, in some cases surgical removal of the affected part of the intestine. Alternative names: regional ileitis, regional enteritis. Oxford Press Concise Medical Dictionary".

It will be of no surprise to those of you who know me well, or have been a patient with this condition, that I do not approve of the items I have put in italics. I found the cause in all cases to be a pancreatic malfunction – the inability of the pancreas to break down specific enzymes going through the alimentary tract by certain foods.

The most common culprits or "triggers" for acute or chronic gut conditions were dairy products, coffee, and cheese, citrus, chocolate. Whole wheat or whole grains were also invariably linked to this condition. It always staggered me that in nearly every case the enterologist or dietician recommended whole wheat and whole bran.

There are various schools of thought as to why whole wheat appears to be a problem. One theory is that the residual pesticides and sprays do not leave the endosperm and create a reaction in the gut. My hypothesis is that the grain is too coarse and enterokinin is produced in the gut and a problem of imbalance ensues. It may well be that both of these probable causes are contributory. Whatever the rights and wrongs may be, I can only speak from the experience of treating hundreds of cases of patients with gut problems and it was resolved by removing all wheat products until the problem was resolved. I supplemented the wheat with white rice, quinoa, cous cous and sago etc; after three weeks, once the bowel had settled down, and there was no sign or blood or mucous I introduced white flour in the shape of bread or pastry. Invariably I also recommended a supplement to replenish and balance the gut flora.

It took on average three weeks for the gut to normalise and for motions to become regular and well formed. The intention must always be to regain balance and to do this one needs to eliminate the "triggers". Provide safe supplementation to boost the immune system and regain balance in the gut. Selenium A-C-E was always a prerequisite along with Colonguard or Enteroguard from Biocare. (Address and phone number at back of book).There were occasions where L-Glutamine or Int B1 were required. Contact your practitioner for advice.

It is absolutely essential to get the supplementation right. I am reminded of a lady who presented with this condition. On testing she was found to be reacting to dairy produce and the 4C syndrome (suspect gut migraine). Coffee, cheese, chocolate, citrus. She had been to see a practitioner local to her who had found her to be reacting to the same things. So a puzzlement – what then was still causing a severe reaction? I then asked if she was taking a supplement from this practitioner – yes, she was. Fortunately she had brought this supplement with her and I could check the ingredients. A major constituent – Bioflavinoids. Unless stated otherwise these are always citrus so beware and read the label. I was not surprised that this lady was getting worse. Once these tablets were removed she settled down very quickly and the gut returned to normal. Practitioners take note please.

Headache and Migraine

Unless you have experienced the debilitation of a migraine headache you will find it hard to imagine the awful pain and nausea that ensues. Those who suffer with migraine describe a feeling of having the head pulled apart in different directions, or of the skull being crushed – of being hypersensitive to bright lights to the point of being restricted to a dark room. Others describe severe nausea and vomiting.

One young man from Frinton on Sea used to have a twice weekly severe migraine, bearing in mind that the effects can last for days; he did not have much of a life, these migraines made him paralysed down the right side. On elimination of the food sensitivities he became paralysed from the neck down and in extreme pain. The parents who were with him at the consultation rang to say how seriously affected he was and asked if they should call a doctor. I advised them not to do so. The reason? With a condition as severe as this there are no short cuts, the bullet must be bitten. Make sure the patient sips water to prevent dehydration. After two days he recovered and slowly returned to normal, and I am delighted to say that apart from one slip up he has been fine.

What was the slip up? He went to his sister's wedding and quite naturally had a piece of wedding cake, it contained citric acid (Lemon) to which he was hypersensitive. The result was a horrendous migraine and that was enough to ensure he never strayed again. I must stress here that eliminating from this or any condition slowly is not advised. Once the testing has been verified within fourteen hours of elimination the symptoms will kick in with a vengeance. You will probably have the worst migraine you have ever had, but, if you carry through it will all pass within seventy two hours and then no more migraine.

Genito-urinary complaints

These include frequency of micturition (urination), cystitis without evidence of infection, frigidity, impotence, prostatitis, vaginitis, thrush, menstrual problems such as PMT (pre-menstrual tension), intermittent menstruation, amenhorrhoea, menhorrhagia etc. Pre-menstrual tension can be accompanied by bloating, depression, skin lesions, spots, swollen breasts, pains in lower abdomen (gut cramp), inter-cyclical bleeding (between periods). All of these can be ameliorated and resolved by *finding the cause* .More later.

Rheumatism and Arthritis

I have always been convinced that arthritis in all its forms is "triggered" by food sensitivity and breakdown of the immune system. There are thousands of patients walking around pain free and leading normal lives today due to dietary application and supplementation. Are there major culprits? Yes. In the case of osteo arthritis dairy products are invariably the cause, rheumatoid is more complicated but more of that later.

Neurological (Mental) conditions

These can manifest themselves in numerous ways – panic attacks, chronic anxiety, depression, hyperactivity, hyperkinesis, ADDS attention deficit disorder syndrome, purposeless violence, short attention span, brain fg, thought disorder, lack of concentration, dyslexia and epilepsy. I know what you are thinking; here he goes again stating that pancreatic malfunction is the cause of all illness. No I am not saying that at all. What I am saying is that in my many years in practice I treated all these conditions successfully with extremely grateful patients, so you see it is not hypothesis. When the body has been under extreme stress for long periods (chronic) and there is definite organ breakdown then of course operative techniques are necessary. But what a pity these conditions were not treated in the early stages then the operation could have been avoided. Hence the object of this book to help you find a practitioner who can diagnose the problem and put you on the road to recovery.

It is my hypothesis that the human body has been subjected to such enormous stressors in a relatively short time frame that it has become unable to adapt, and adaptogens are an important part of the immune system response. Think of the various additional stressors of recent years – excitotoxins, radiation, pollution, more toxic chemical plants, more pesticides and sprays, the leaching of natural minerals from the soil, preservatives, colourings and additives in food. To cap it all the massive increase of sugar and salt in our food. The average consumption of sugar per person in this country is 48-54 lbs (24 kilos) a year. None of my household takes sugar and neither do many of my friends. So where does it go? Is it really surprising that diabetes is on the increase? The pancreas is incapable of coping with these large amounts and the liver is unable to cope with the excessive fats in food.

If an engine is designed to run on different fuels then the component parts need to be structurally altered to run smoothly on that type of fuel. The body would need to go through the slow evolutionary process taking millennia to adapt to what it is expected to cope with today.

Why am I referring to this action when referring to neurological/mental conditions? For two reasons. One is that very few people realise that something wrong with the brain functioning correctly has a connection with the instigatory organ – the pancreas. If you doubt this statement then I suggest very strongly that you read Brain Allergies the Psychonutrient Connection by Kalita and Philpott now available in paperback.*It will help you to understand how the pancreas affects the brain but the need to have proper supplementation to repair the immune system – balance! **See recommended reading page.*

Homoeostasis

Some time ago I was having a discussion with my friend the GP

Dr Andrew Tresidder who wrote the foreword to this book, and amongst his other attributes is an expert on flower remedies, he was saying that it is rare to find a patient who understands the concept of balance; the spiritual, physical and emotional and getting the balance right. How right he was. How can the mind be crystal clear if it is being polluted? How can your central computer (pancreas) function correctly if it is being compromised by a wrong ingestion of food? How can we aspire to spirituality if there is no peace within? If our systems are in turmoil, the immune system being continually bombarded and weakened, the adrenal glands under stress, it is impossible to achieve homoeostasis – ***balance.*** To contact Dr Tresidder www.drandrew.co.uk.

Our bodies are a miracle of complexities and to understand the concept it is advisable to consider it as a piece of delicate and incredibly complicated machinery. In this day and age the one piece of machinery everyone seems to have is a computer and you will know that the slightest mistake, a full stop or comma in the wrong place it will not respond. The adage that I believe originated in the USA is apt. ***Rubbish in – rubbish out!*** Our bodies are no different; if you feed one piece of wrong information in (food or drink) you will not get the right response. The pancreas – our central computer will malfunction. The enzymatic processes instigated by the pancreas are "scrambled" and in turn the adrenal glands, the kidneys, spleen, liver and brain are scrambled too – garbage out!

The Mechanism of Allergic Reaction

It would be remiss of me not to try and explain to you the mechanism of allergic reaction. A person who is allergic will react to his or her allergen in rather the same way a healthy person reacts to a dangerous toxin or micro-organism. In both cases the body's defences are stimulated by the presence of an antigen (living or organic matter foreign to our own proteins).

Viruses and bacteria are antigens, and so are normally less dangerous substances like food, pollens etc; our defences depend and rely on lymphocytes (white cells) whose function is to distinguish between harmful and innocuous antigens. When white cells are alerted to an antigen, which looks as though it may cause harm to the body, they produce antibodies. The antibodies combine with the antigens and render it harmless.

Even in a healthy person it may take several days for the white cells to produce enough antibodies to inactivate the antigen. But once the antigen has been dealt with the body has long lasting protection against it. This is possibly why diseases like measles and chickenpox are only generally caught once in their lives. When the virus attacks for the second time there are antibodies at hand to recognise and dispose of it quickly. This is the general idea behind vaccination, you are given a minute dose of an antigen which is not strong enough to give you the disease but is strong enough to activate the white cells and protect you. However, it is generally accepted that the common cold or similar should not be vaccinated against.

In an allergy prone person the white cells react to a harmless antigen as if it were an invader. No one is really clear why this should happen, although evidence indicates that it may well be a hereditary problem. Allergies do tend to run in families and there is some evidence that allergic people lack a particular set of white cells that controls the production of antibodies. It certainly appears to be more prevalent in children who have not been breast fed or weaned off the bottle too soon and leaving them prone to infection later in their lives. This often reveals itself as an allergy to cow's milk and dairy products. This tendency is further complicated by the fact that we have not one, but several mechanisms for allergic reactions.

Certainly it became apparent to me throughout my practice life, that children removed from the breast immediately, or after a short space of time were more prone to early breakdown of the immune system. It is my hypothesis that the immunoglobulin IgE and possibly IgA were the hereditary factor. I found that the trend in 97.5 % of cases that it was passed from mother to son, and father to daughter. IgE and IgA are part of a group of structurally related proteins that act as antibodies. Several classes of immunoglobulins with differing functions are IgE, IgA, IgG, IgD and IgM.

What usually happens?

That depends entirely on where the mast cells are located. As I have mentioned earlier in the description of "the Stress Syndrome", we are compartmentalised like a ship. If the mast cells affected are in the head then symptoms like nasal catarrh, streaming nose, headache or migraine. In the chest compartment – persistent irritating cough, asthma, bronchitis. In the gut compartment – constipation, bowel cramps, diarrhoea, Crohn's disease.

Our biological structures are all different, just like our fingerprints. So the problem facing a practitioner specialising in allergy/food sensitivity reactions (Clinical Ecologist) are enormous and hugely complicated. Hence the reason for writing this book. A good analogy would be that of crossing a minefield. But over all those years in practice a pattern did emerge – certain symptoms fell in to a certain food category and I have become even more aware of this since I retired and have had more time to study the subject. I am therefore hoping that by writing this book I will be able to save many hundreds of people from unnecessary suffering.

Nothing is ever 100% foolproof but I am confident that if you follow the advice given there will be an improvement in your condition. There is no doubt that some symptoms will need further investigation and this why you should consult your doctor first. Then if there is a possibility of a serious problem you will be referred to a specialist. When it has been fully investigated and it is proven that there is no serious underlying cause, then, and only then before you consider taking any drug or drugs, which all have side effects, you can then try the procedures I suggest. Light the blue touch paper and stand back in amazement.

Methods of Testing for Allergy

The elimination method

This is a long drawn out procedure that can last for weeks. When the symptoms are multi-factorial it is almost impossible to determine the cause. If you decide to take this course of action then simplify your diet as much as possible. Lamb, potato, calabrese (broccoli) as a main meal and pear as fruit. Later you will see an elimination diet sheet which is 1,000 calories a day and should help with elimination of toxins. Be prepared to feel worse before you feel better. The body does not like changing patterns and loves to hold on to what has become "the norm". Are there typical withdrawal symptoms? Everyone is different but the most common are as follows: - headache, nausea, shakiness, perspiration, clamminess, aching in all joints, raised or lowered pulse rate and influenza type symptoms. These can last up to three to five days.

It really is amazing the spectrum one hear from patients. They vary from "I don't know why you made all that fuss, I did not feel a thing" to "You were quite right to warn me I thought I was going to die". It is impossible to say where you will fall in that spectrum, but a good rule of thumb is – if your symptoms have been severe and chronic then the chances are your initial reaction could be quite bad. Mild symptoms usually induce a mild response. I recall some years ago telling a lady in a wheelchair crippled with arthritis –"You will almost certainly have quite serious withdrawal symptoms and they could last for as long as three weeks. This is normal, take your painkillers and once the pain and swelling have gone you will feel so much better". Well, how wrong can you be? Three weeks later I had a phone call from this lady "where is all this pain and discomfort you said I would have, I am out of my wheelchair doing the washing up at the kitchen sink?" I explained that she had been incredibly lucky and her type of recovery was not "the norm" and her pain must have been so bad that she did not notice the change.

Conversely I remember a gentleman from Chepstow with gout which seriously affected his feet and ankles. I told him that he may have pain and discomfort for a few days but it should clear very quickly. The poor chap was on the phone to me every week for six weeks in absolute agony and unable to put his feet to the floor. He crawled everywhere. I begged him not to give up on the way of eating I had suggested and he agreed to give it another week, thankfully six weeks and three days later he was free of pain and was able to put his shoes on for the first time in six weeks. Thankfully he has not had a moment's problem since. So, you will see from the contrast in these two patients no matter how good a practitioner you are, surprises will occur. What it does prove is that the diagnosis was correct and the way of eating recommended was the right one. But, always advise the patient of what could happen.

The "scratch" test

This is a simple test in which an area of healthy skin is selected and cleansed with alcohol, and then a tiny, painless scratch with a sterile needle is made. The scratch is so light that no blood is drawn; a drop of the allergen is placed on the skin and left for fifteen to thirty minutes, then wiped off. If the area has become inflamed and irritable then a positive reaction is recorded. As many as one hundred tests could be carried out at one sitting but this would be most unusual.

The Intradermal test

The intradermal test gets its name from the fact that allergen is dissolved in liquid and injected in to the skin. Another area of skin, in close proximity to the first, is then selected and clear liquid injected. It is then possible to compare the two for any redness or swelling which would indicate an allergic reaction. The intradermal test is often used because it gives a quicker reaction. The results can be read in a time scale from eight to fifteen minutes. Like the scratch test it is not painful but must be administered with care.

The Patch Test

An area of skin is cleansed with alcohol and a piece of gauze is dipped in the suspected allergen and then taped on to the skin. Checks can be made at regular intervals to observe any inflammation or irritation in the area. The gauze can be left on for as long as three days to determine a reaction. However, if there is a strong reaction then it would be removed immediately and the area swabbed off.

The Eye Test

Should you be one of the many patients who react violently to allergenic substances then the eye test may be used. The reactions to this test are similar. A drop of the suspected substance is placed in the corner of the eye and ten to fifteen minutes later the eye is carefully examined for any redness or irritation. The substance may cause the patient to sneeze violently, indicating an allergic reaction. The symptoms usually wear off after thirty minutes but can take as long as two hours.

The Davies Test

There is little doubt in my mind that the method I have been using for over thirty years, with 100% repetition, is not, and probably never will be accepted as scientific, it has proved to be the most effective and painless method I have come across. It is by far the most effective way of the patient knowing immediately their sensitivities. It is Applied or Clinical Kinesiology – the inter-reaction between the musculature and various organs of the body. I should point out the previous tests mentioned have all been external reactions the Davies method is an internal response. The most common foods used for testing are the ones usually used in every day households. Milk, butter, cheese, sugar, egg yolk, egg white, citrus fruit, coffee, tea, white flour, whole wheat flour, nuts, tomato and chocolate.

The substance is placed under the tongue on to the sub-lingual and sub-mandibular glands. These have an immediate response with the pancreas, the instigatory endocrine/exocrine organ of the body. Our central computer. That nerve reflex controls and supports the latissimus dorsii, teres minor and the triceps muscles. The patient is placed on the couch with a raised, adjustable back, so that they are in a semi-reclining position. The arm is placed with the elbow resting on the hip bone and the forearm bent to an angle of just below 90 degrees, hand and wrist held firm and pointing upwards. The substance is then placed under the tongue and a pressure of approx 3-5lbs (1.4 – 2.2 kilos) is applied with thumb on to the patient's wrist. The patient is then told to resist the pressure, which should always be across the gut line. If the pressure is withheld then no reaction. However if the patient cannot resist that pressure and the arm collapses across the gut line then there is a positive reaction. Both patient and practitioner are immediately aware of the effect. I must remind you that the bent arm should be at an angle of 80 degrees and not 90 degrees as this will bring the biceps in to play and ruin the test.

It is important at this juncture to make it clear that neither the sub-lingual test nor the muscle test are inventions of mine. Muscle testing is down to Dr George Goodheart. Dr Guy Pfeiffer and Dr Lawrence D. Dickey were responsible for refining the sub-lingual procedure around 1962. Their methodology was different to mine. The substance was placed under the tongue because the veins under the tongue are close to the surface and react readily in absorbing traces of foods, drinks, and drugs. (This is why heart stimulating drugs such as nitro-glycerine are placed under the tongue for immediate absorption). A careful procedure of taking the patient's pulse at rest , then placing the substance under the tongue and checking for any marked fluctuation in pulse rate, pupil size, facial colour, respiration etc were monitored and carefully notated. Dr Arthur Coca refined this even further calling it the Coca Test, and if there was more than 12 beats variation in pulse rate a reaction was positive. This method whilst very accurate was by necessity time consuming and because the substances were left under the tongue, were deleterious to the patient's health.

Dr Richard Mackarness in his excellent book *Not All In the Mind,* describes the techniques used and was certainly responsible for bringing to the attention of the medical profession in this country, and the public at large, that an alternative method of food sensitivity testing was possible and effective. I thought long and hard about these methods and was fortunately invited to a seminar in Devon on Applied Kinesiology by Brian H. Butler. He was a brilliant instructor and I learnt much from him. I certainly owe him a debt of gratitude. It was after many months of studying these techniques that I became aware that certain muscle groups also affected certain nerve reflexes. I experimented on friends and family for many months until I was convinced that it was repeatable procedure. Hence the Davies test was born and the subsequent decades have proved how effective it has been.

I would like to intersperse patient's letters throughout this book, totally unsolicited, so that it will encourage you to adopt the methods outlined in this book or to have a consultation with a Clinical Ecologist.

Dear Mr Davies,

I am writing to let you know that I will not be needing my second appointment. There is a very good reason for me not to attend and that is that I finally believe I have got rid of the dreadful allergy that has been ruining my life for the last five years.

Thanks to your wonderful technique, knowledge and most of all your positive attitude, my husband and I can begin to lead a normal life again. As I mentioned to you during our session we had spent a considerable amount of money on seeing various dermatologists in Bristol to find a cure for my allergy. The symptoms were, as my husband put it, "like someone putting a blowtorch over your face".

As you know, these "Professionals" could not come up with any helpful suggestions and it made us quite ill to have to pay bills! After my consultation with you I went home and started the recommended diet, a little dubious I must confess. After all, we had already tried conventional methods and failed, so why should this be any different?

Since the day I left your office I have not had a serious attack. The only time the allergy returns is when I have strayed off the diet and even then it is not bad because I am not poisoning myself with the wrong foods on a daily basis. We are expecting our first baby in August as you know, and now I no longer have to contend with the misery of the allergy. At last I am blooming!

So thank you again Mr Davies for such a simple and effective remedy and I know that if any of our friends or relations become ill through allergies they will be coming to see you!

Yours sincerely

A.B. Bristol.

The object of printing these letters, and the originals are here for inspection at any time, is to point out the simplicity of the test, the speed of recovery, and the need to comply with the restrictions placed upon you by the results of the tests. As mentioned in the previous letter and in others in the book you will understand how committed you have to be. If you wander from the "straight and narrow" then you suffer unnecessarily. If you cheat, you only cheat one person – yourself! I have used a saying for decades with my patients and it is one that will always hold true –"Your body is the church in which you worship – how you worship is entirely up to you".

The Pancreas

This is the instigatory endocrine/exocrine organ/gland in the body; a compound gland, about 15cm long, that lies behind the stomach. One end lies in the curve of the duodenum, the other touches the spleen. It is composed of clusters (acini) of cells that secrete pancreatic juice. These contain a number of enzymes concerned in digestion. The juice drains into small ducts that open in to the pancreatic duct. This unites with the common bile duct and the secretions pass in to the duodenum.

Interspersed among the acini are the Islets of Langerhans – an isolated group of cells that secrete the hormones insulin and glucagon in to the bloodstream. Insulin regulates the metabolism of carbohydrates and controls the blood sugar level. A deficiency in the production of insulin results in *diabetes mellitus*, commonly referred to as sugar diabetes, the condition in which the body is unable to use its blood sugar, which then builds up in the blood and is required to be excreted by the kidneys. This state is called hyperglycaemia.

By distinction, the over activity of insulin through dietary transgressions removes glucose from the blood by increased combustion and enlarges the store of glycogen at the expense of the glucose. This state is called hypoglycaemia. Since the brain depends on a constant supply of glucose, sufferers can pass out, with clamminess, sudden loss of energy, hunger, and in extreme cases epileptic seizures and collapse.

As you will see by the explanation above how vital it is that the pancreas is functioning correctly. It is our central computer and like all computers if you feed one piece of wrong information in you will get wrong information out, or, the system will not work at all. The whole of my practice life was based on this fact and the success I achieved with my patients was due to correcting any malfunction taking place. What is the one thing that we do every day of our lives? We eat and drink. If we eat or drink the wrong things then it is not surprising that a pancreatic malfunction occurs.

Hippocrates the father of modern medicine coined a phrase which has been translated in to "We are what we eat". I have read many transcriptions of his sayings, and I am fairly sure that the literal translation was in fact "Look in your food cupboard before you look in your drug cupboard". Regardless of the merits of the translation what this incredibly knowledgeable man was saying in effect was, put the right fuel in and the system will function correctly. Let's be sensible about this, if you went to the local garage to put fuel in your car would you put the wrong fuel in. Of course you wouldn't. So, why treat our incredibly complicated engine any differently?

The tests we carried out were performed in my clinic. The tests were carried out with sole intention of the patient being informed of the whole process. The testing, the finding of allergens, the elimination of those, the possible withdrawal symptoms and the outcome of the continuous ingestion of toxic substances. In other words carried out in a controlled environment. If you have any adverse symptomology then always consult your doctor first. They will ascertain whether the problem is organic or not and advise accordingly. Having said that, if you have exhausted all the normal procedures and are being told – "there is nothing wrong with you, all tests show negative, you must learn to live with it" then, and only then, find a Clinical Ecologist or consider the alternatives I am setting out for you in this book.

Reintroducing allergenic substances

I was always amused by the difference in attitude between my German patients and us "Brits". Remembering of course that their chemists are split in to two sections, allopathic and homoeopathic, so they always have had options. But their attitude once they were told the sensitivities that they had was "ok doc I will stick with it and if it is for life, so be it". Our attitude is different. Almost as soon as the symptoms have gone patients are saying "when can I go back on the suspect foods". As it is usually the case that patient's problems are chronic (long term), then it is fairly obvious that the immune system is not going to repair overnight. It will take at least three months so don't rush it. Even then it is only if the vital "balance – homeostasis" has been achieved that it could be considered.

The one thing that has to be fully understood is that the base allergens/sensitivities will remain forever, and never to be reintroduced. Where what I call peripheral sensitivities are concerned that is a different kettle of fish and addressed accordingly. Let me explain. If you have suffered with horrendous migraines for many years on a weekly basis great care would be needed. On testing let us assume that you were allergic to dairy produce and the 4c syndrome (now the 3C syndrome, more later). Coffee, citrus, cheese, chocolate and suspect hazelnuts and tomato. Once the migraines have completely gone for three months, then you could try the tomato, if after three days there is no reaction try it again, but not in large quantities. If the adrenal glands are functioning correctly and no reaction has taken place then try the hazelnuts a few at a time. You could carry out a simple Coca test when you have ingested the suspect food. Sit quietly for ten minutes, take your pulse. If steady then eat the suspect food and sit quietly again for twenty minutes, then check the pulse, thirty minutes after that check the pulse again, if there is a fluctuation of 12 beats up or down then you know there is a reaction. Take a teaspoonful of bi-carbonate of soda, in a cup of warm water and sip slowly. This will prevent any serious reaction.

It is possible for dramatic reactions to occur. I am reminded of a lady who presented with urticaria (hives), which amongst other things produced a marked swelling and wheals on her hands. When she returned six weeks later all signs of the condition had disappeared. However – over the festive season she had a glass of sherry and her comments were as follows; - "I could not believe my eyes, within ten minutes both my hands were red, swollen and painful". That is a case where the bi-carb would have helped.

Another classic case was experienced by my first publisher. He had suffered with migraines for years. We tested him and it was the 4C syndrome again. He excluded them and had a nasty few days' withdrawal but great relief – no more migraine. Bearing in mind what I had told him about reintroduction after three months he had a coffee and got away with it. So he continued having the occasional coffee with no problem. He rang and told me he was coming down from London to Taunton and would I meet him at the station. Of course I did so, but when the train pulled in no immediate sign of him, then he appeared getting off the train very gingerly and saying "are you there Gwynne?", I walked hurriedly toward him and it soon became evident that he could not focus correctly. He had a blinding migraine. He told me what he had done. While waiting for the departure of his train he had a coffee. But when on the train he bought a bar of chocolate and ate it. Well! That was too much for the adrenal glands and the mast cells so the reaction was severe. He never did that again.

The importance of diet and nutrition has been slipping slowly into the sunset, but, as with fashion, things are slowly coming round again. Organic food is now far more available in supermarkets. Schools of Medicine are giving doctor's six hours of training in four years. I know, it is a pin prick, but in the right direction. In their splendid book *Brain Allergies – The*

Psychonutrient and Magnetic Connection Kalita and Philpott refer continually to the importance of pancreatic function and state "the pancreas is the first endocrine/exocrine organ influenced by ingested food and chemicals. It has the monumental task of buffering against reaction to any of these substances". In his book *How to Control Your Allergies,* Robert Forman PhD devotes a whole chapter to hypoglycaemia, allergy and the pancreas.

So, you will see by now that the testing I carried out in my clinic for over thirty years, and the remarkable results we achieved were absolutely correct. Hopefully through this book I will enable and encourage you to take the steps toward good health and happiness.

The following was sent to me by a patient many years ago, I have no idea who composed it, but it is as true today as it was all those years ago.

A Cautionary Tale

Little Pete would only eat
Packaged puddings very sweet
Fizzy drinks with tartrazine
Pork pies and pastries filled with cream
He ignored his parent's desperate pleas
To eat vegetables, fruit and cheese
They keep him propped up in the hall
As a warning to you all not to share their young son's fate
Who perished before his sell by date
For his cravings for E200's tabooed
Any sort of healthy food
They noticed with alarm
His legs had started to embalm
As the process reached his chin
Still little Pete would not give in
And at the end his cry was ***never***
Now little Pete's preserved for ever.
Anonymous

Here to finish this chapter is a "good news" letter.

Chepstow
Gwent
Dear Mr Davies,
About nine years ago I came to you with health problems that had been with me for several years, headaches, palpitations, digestion problems etc:

My own doctor had been of little help. But after cutting out cow's milk, white flour, citrus, coffee etc; as you instructed, the results after a few weeks were truly amazing. My health over the past nine years has been wonderful, no headaches or previous problems at all. I am very fit indeed, doing a lot of competitive running which I always loved before my health problems; in fact, I have never felt better!

I am so very grateful to you and cannot thank you enough; it really changed my life.

Yours sincerely
M.M. (Male)

Chapter 2

Which Foods Are at Fault

In my first book *Overcoming Food Allergies* I made a comment at the beginning of Chapter 2 about not blaming any particular food industry, and that statement still holds good. I am not blaming any one particular industry out of hand; there are criticisms that can be offered about many aspects of the food industry in general and the advertising of food. The manufacture of food. How organic is organic food? But one industry and their products became so evident in as many as 95% of the cases I saw in over thirty years, and that was the dairy industry and associated products, lactose, lactic acid, casein and whey. I would like to quote from an independent newspaper article that appeared some years ago but is as pertinent today.

> *New research suggests that for some, milk can be responsible for chronic disease and general ill- health. It can even affect a child's handwriting and lead to allegations of child maltreatment. Each year we get through several billion litres of milk. It is promoted as a healthy drink, full of goodness, but for many it is also a health problem, and researchers are questioning the wisdom of drinking so much. Milk marketing organisations have promoted the value of milk for health and fitness to such an extent that the medical and nursing professions, as well as the general public, have become convinced that milk is good for you. The idea that milk can also be very bad for you has become almost heresy and the fact that cow's milk was intended for baby cow's, not for baby humans, seems to have been forgotten – says Dr Harry Morrow Brown, the Derbyshire based physician and allergist.*

Milk and cheese consumption may also be responsible for the increase in prostate and testicular cancers in the UK and other western countries. Researchers from the Medical University of Yamanashi in Japan looked at the cancer rates and diet in 42 countries and found significant links between cheese and testicular cancer, and milk and prostate cancer. They found that those with a high consumption of dairy products also had high rates of cancers. The UK with a testicular cancer rate of 13 per 100,000 had a cheese consumption of 12 grams a day. In Algeria, with a zero rate for the cancer, cheese consumption was less than three grams a day.

Other teams of researchers have found links between milk and a range of other diseases and health problems including insulin dependent diabetes. This has fuelled claims that cow's milk is not a natural food for humans. As I have already pointed out 95% of cases that tested for anything from brittle nails to cancer, had an allergic reaction to dairy. Michelle Berriedale-Johnson, the editor of Inside Story, a journal for people on a restrictive diet said, *"We are the only mammal that continues to drink milk of any kind after weaning and certainly the only one that drinks the milk of another species. People in the Far East are naturally lactose intolerant, but due to the Americanisation of their diet they are learning to tolerate lactose"*. It is also of great interest that Professor Jane Plant in her excellent book *Your Life in Your Hands – Understanding, Preventing and Overcoming Breast Cancer* found that when she researched the fact so few cases of breast cancer occurred in China, it was the fact that so few of them ever touched dairy products. If anyone reading this book needs to be made aware of the link between dairy and cancer, particularly breast and testicular cancer, I would strongly recommend that you read her book.

Within days of the article in the Independent newspaper an article appeared in one of the tabloid newspapers about a baby of five months that was registered at a nursery, the parents insistingon numerous occasions that their baby was allergic to cow's milk etc; a nursery nurse fed her a breakfast cereal which clearly stated that it contained milk protein. The baby died. This was a severe reaction and she died of anaphylactic shock. This reaction certainly does not always become this severe. But, in my vast experience, once you have been found intolerant to dairy products you would be wise to avoid them completely. The ingestion of same will put immense strain on your immune system. So the answer is simple, particularly in those with heart problems – leave well alone and be extremely vigilant.

I am reminded of a lady patient who came from Bridgwater Somerset. She was only 30 years of age, and on her first visit I watched her ease her way slowly and painfully up the stairs, with the help of her husband. She asked me not to shake her hand as they were so swollen and painful. Her doctor had diagnosed her nine months earlier with arthritis. She was quite tearful and told me that being so young, she did not want to "live with it", or live on drugs for the rest of her life. Taking her case history the following symptomology was manifested:- severe swelling of hands, knees and feet, total fatigue, chronic constipation (common in arthritis), pre-menstrual tension and menses very light, panic attacks and chronic anxiety and depression brought about by the sudden onset of severe pain and deformative swellings. Her allergies/sensitivities followed an all too familiar pattern – milk, butter, cheese, white flour, orange, tomato, rhubarb, gooseberry, strawberry, beetroot, spinach, peppers, radish, and apple skin.

On her return visit six weeks later she ran up the stairs looking radiant and said " I really don't know why I am here, I feel absolutely wonderful – thank you so much". On questioning I found that all of her previous symptomology had disappeared. It would not be unheard of that when she returned to her doctor and told him what had happened, in all probability she would be told that she was in remission and be prepared for it to return. I wish I had a pound for every time I have heard this said. It certainly appears that main stream medicine will not accept that food sensitivity does exist. Knowing this could be the reaction I took the precaution of checking up on this lady many years later and, like many hundreds of others she was symptom free.

Why milk? It would be far more acceptable if there were a sensible straightforward answer. It is so complicated that to my knowledge no one is really sure why so many of us react to dairy products. The easiest explanation and the most simplistic is that we were never meant to ingest a food meant for another species. Admittedly goat and sheep milk are tolerated better than cow's milk if you are lactose intolerant then these are a non starter. Soya (organic) or rice milk or oat milk are alternatives.

The enzymes required to break down and digest milk are rennin and lactase. By the age of four many of us lose the ability to digest lactose because we can no longer synthesize the digestive enzyme lactase. This lactose intolerance results in diarrhoea, flatulence and bowel or stomach cramps. Some 90% of adult Asian and coloured people and 20% of Caucasian children are lactose intolerant. The level of the protein casein in cow's milk is 300 times higher than in human breast milk, which is predominantly made up of the protein lactalbumin which is easily digestible by babies.

Nature has designed the milk of each animal species specifically to suit the needs of its young. Casein is intended to be broken down by the four stomach digestive system of baby calves. In human stomachs it coagulates and forms large, tough, dense and difficult to digest curds. When protein of another animal is introduced in to the body it may cause an allergic reaction (*Journal of Allergy,41.226.1968),* the most common symptom of which are runny nose (rhinitis), persistent sore throat, hoarseness, bronchitis and recurrent ear infections. The mucus membranes lining the joints and lungs can become swollen and inflamed contributing to asthma and rheumatoid arthritis of which more later in the book).

One of the most outspoken opponents of dairy products, and there are many both here in the UK and in the United States is Dr William A. Ellis and he states; "Over my 42 years in practice I have performed more than 25,000 blood tests for my patients. These tests show conclusively, in my opinion, that adults who use milk do not absorb nutrients as well as the patients who do not. Of course, poor absorption, in turn, means chronic fatigue". Obviously I am going to concur with this observation. As I have stated already 95% of the thousands of patients I have tested have been hypersensitive to cow's milk. Milk is touted as a great natural source of calcium. We need it for healthy teeth and bones and it prevents osteoporosis. In fact ingesting dairy products can increase the rate at which calcium is lost from the body and so hasten osteoporosis. As well as being high in calcium, dairy products are also high in protein. If we have too much protein in the diet from milk products or any other source, such as meat, fish or eggs the body is required to eliminate the excess. To do this the kidneys must lose calcium as they cleanse the blood of excess waste, a process known as protein induced hypercalcuria *(J.Nutr,III:553,1981:Trans NY Acad Sci 36:333,1974:Am Clin Nutr 27:916,1974)*

I will ask you one question – the largest animal on earth is the elephant with strong bones, enormous tusks and yet I have never seen one drink milk. Have you? The body's ability to absorb and utilise calcium depends on the amount of phosphorous in our diet. The higher the proportion of phosphorous to calcium the less the bone loss and consequently a stronger skeletal system, providing the intake protein is not high. The foods that contain higher phosphorous/calcium ratios are fruit and vegetables. Low fat milk is no better as it contains 1% butterfat and a full complement of allergy inciting milk protein.

To the list of problems naturally inherent in human consumption of milk designed for baby calves we can add a whole host of unnatural ones. Cow's milk contains the residues of accumulated antibiotics, pesticides and sprays in the grain fed to cattle, the female hormones given to cow's to increase the yield and their body fat. Some milk has also been shown to contain trace metals and radioactivity at levels higher than those permissible in drinking water. Back in my practice days the milk produced in America was contaminated with leukaemia viruses, at that time it was 20% - this has now increased considerably, and any of you who have read Professor Freed's book on milk will be aware how that contamination can affect the whole pool of milk when collected in the bulk tanks.

The cancer inducing viruses are resistant to being killed by pasteurisation, as are many parasites, and they have been recovered from supermarket supplies. Is it beyond belief that the highest rates of leukaemia are found in children aged 3-13 who consume the most milk products and dairy farmers who, as a profession, have the highest rates of leukaemia for any occupational group.

The book I have recommended by Professor David Freed, Bailliere Tindall 1984, called *Health Hazards of Milk* is not freely available but it really does contain everything you need to know about the ingestion of cow's milk. I hope by outlining the problems involved you will understand that toward the end of my practice life I took everyone off cow's milk as a precautionary measure.

Foods Containing Milk

Baking powder
Biscuits
Bakers bread
Bavarian cream
Blancmange
Boiled salad dressings
Bologna
Butter
Fritters
Gravies
Hash
Hard sauces
Ice cream
Malted milk
Ovaltine
Meat loaf

Buttermilk
Butter sauces
Cakes
Chocolates
Chocolate or cocoa drinks
Cream
Creamed foods
Cream sauces
Cheeses
Curds
Custards
Eggs scrambled
Escalloped dishes
Food prepared au gratin
Food fried in butter
Flour mixtures
Sausages
Milk chocolate
Milk in all forms
Oleomargarines
Pie crust made with milk products
Popcorn
Popovers
Prepared mixes for cake making or biscuits
Doughnuts, muffins, pancakes, pie crust
Waffles and puddings
Rarebit
Sherbets
Souffles
Soups
Sweets

In other words we are back to the old maxim – **check the labels on all foodstuffs.**

White flour

I cannot tell you how thankful I am that today it is possible to obtain white flour and bread organically in all shops and supermarkets. To my intense delight the government and the flour industry have seen fit to exclude the 52 additives and preservatives that were in white flour for many years.

Why do I bother to mention this fact? For a very good reason. It is general medical opinion that many inexplicable symptoms are occurring – flu viruses are mutating – superbugs are now rife throughout the country – cot death syndrome became prevalent but is now under control – neurological diseases appear to be on the increase – so why are these things happening? Why is cancer in all its forms, other than leukaemia, on the increase? There are very few families that are not affected by this scourge. I ask you to remember one thing at this moment – the above paragraph was written in my last book in 2004 – nothing has changed and if anything it has worsened. Is it possible that ingesting 52 additives and preservatives to the very "staff of life" (flour) attacked and weakened the immune system of the nation? It is a well known and documented fact that propionates induce cancer – but at least four were used in bread making!

It is also a well known medical fact that drugs can contra indicate (fight each other), and so can foods and food, and foods and drugs. How much attention is paid to this? I suspect not a lot. At the risk of stating the obvious I will list the ingredients that were in white flour. You may require help, as you are not an industrial chemist, and I am pleased to tell you that help is at hand should you need it. *Foresight – the Organisation for Pre-conceptual Care* produces two excellent booklets with all the E-Numbers in and a booklet containing toxins in food. I would recommend you to obtain these and I will give you their address in the appendix.

E150 Caramel	E170 Calcium carbonate
E220 Sulphur dioxide	E221 Sodium sulphite
E222 Sodium hydrogen sulphate	E223 Sodium metabisulphate
E224 Potassium metabisulphate	E226 Calcium sulphite
E227 Calcium hydrogen sulphite	E260 Acetic acid
E262 Sodium hydrogen diacetate	E270 Lactic acid
E280 Propionic acid	E281 Sodium propionate
E282 Calcium propionate	E283 Potassium propionate

E290 Carbon dioxide
E300 Ascorbic acid
E322 Lecithin
E330 Citric acid
E333 Tricalcium citrate
E336 Monopotassium L-tartrate
E341 Calcium tetrahydrogen
E450 Disodium dihydrogen diphosphate
E460 Alpha-cellulose
E450 Ethylmethylcellulose
E446 Carboxymethylcellulose sodium salt
E471 Mono and di-glycerides of fatty acids
E472b Lactic acid esters of mono and
E472c Citric acid esters of mono and di-Di-glycerides fatty acids. Glycerides of fatty acids
E472e Mono-and diacetyltartaric
E481 Sodium stearoyl 2 lactylate
E482 Calcium stearoyl 2 lactylate
E483 Stearyl tartrate
500 Sodium hydrogen carbonate
510 Ammonium chloride
516 Calcium sulphate
541 Sodium aluminium phosphate acidic
641 D-glucono -1,5 lactone
920 L-cysteine hydrochloride
924 Potassium bromate
925 Chlorine
926 Chlorine dioxide
927 Azodicarbonamide
Ammonium dihydrogen orthophosphate
Diammonium hydrogen orthophosphate
Ammonium chloride
Calcium sulphate
Amylases
Proteinases
Nitrogen
Benzoyl peroxide

I would be willing to bet that you now feel totally enriched. I find that list mind boggling and it might just as well be in Chinese or Greek. You can see by this list that manufacturers use gobbledygook to sell their products to the general public, my burning question is still, and always has been, why on earth was this Frankenstein monster allowed to burgeon from simple flour as used by the French, to this monstrous concoction?

Fine, it no longer exists, but for how many years was this chemical concoction allowed to be part of the staple diet of the British public? At least 15 years and you can imagine what it did to the gut flora in the process. Wheat before milling is treated with benzoyl peroxide as a bleaching agent. Traces of this remain after the processing and are a primary cause of allergy/food sensitivity. You are strongly advised not to use bleached packet breads and where possible use organic.

In my first book *Overcoming Food Allergies*, I used the axiom *"the whiter the bread the quicker your dead"*. Proponents of white flour will tell you it is better than wholemeal because it is "enriched" – minerals and vitamins added back in to it. When I see that word I am reminded of the story Abram Hoffer tells in his book *Orthomolecular Nutrition* when this subject is aired. "You are walking along a street and a mugger pulls a gun on you and orders you to strip naked. The thief takes your clothes and valuables. Noticing your shivering embarrassment he returns your underclothes and gives you fifty pence to catch the bus home. Do you feel enriched"?

One young lady who did not feel enriched came to see me some years ago. I will call her Wendy, she was 18 years of age and accompanied by her mother. Thank goodness mother was there – I could not get one word out of Wendy. She just sat there with her chin resting on her chest, her eyes cast down towards the floor and looking extremely pale and totally disinterested in anything I was saying. It was obvious that she was not well but how was I going to get through to her? I did not wish to bring mother in as the spokesperson but there was no option and the conversation went as follows:-

GHD	What is wrong with your daughter, she does not look well?
MOTHER	No, she is not well and yet she is not ill as such. From the age of thirteen she slowly retracted in to her shell, not interested in going out, no school, tired all the time – in fact a zombie.
GHD	Has she been like this all the time, or is it just moodiness?
MOTHER	No, I don't think it is moods, just total withdrawal from the real world.
GHD	I will ask you some questions to see if any of the symptoms sound like Wendy's.

I then started with the case history questionnaire. There certainly appeared to be nothing organically wrong with Wendy – so was there a pancreatic malfunction? It looked as though Wendy was being hormonally challenged or was slowly being poisoned. I tested her and found her to be totally hypersensitive to white flour and sugar. I warned mother that the withdrawal symptoms could be traumatic and things could get worse before getting better. In fact Wendy came through with flying colours, no real problems, and getting better as each day passed. Three weeks later she went for a holiday in Spain with friends and a few months later applied for and secured a job as a groom in Austria. She kept in touch for years and is enjoying life to the full.

This is just one example of the insidious nature of a product that creates a pancreatic malfunction. But it is my hypothesis that the sudden emergence of *Myalgic encephalomyelitis* (yuppie flu) *was* no coincidence at that time. It resulted in many university students and high flyers in the City of London succumbing to "wipe out" and losing valuable time as a result. Thankfully those who consulted me recovered very quickly once we discovered the causator "trigger".

Wendy's mum was furious when she realised what had caused her daughter's decline and lobbied her member of parliament and others in serious positions who would listen – but to no avail. As this was the case I was determined to help in any way that I could. Needless to say I will not be mentioning names but two prominent members of both Houses of Parliament brought their children to see me, both children far from well. This gave me the ideal opportunity to "climb on my soap box" and give them my opinion on the insidious nature of foods like white flour etc. I did not have much hope of achieving anything but felt better for airing my very strong views. So, you can imagine my surprise when I was informed that the Prime Minister of the day had ordered the elimination of additives and preservatives in white flour production some three months later. Incredibly – Wendy was the catalyst for a major change in government policy.

Ask yourself this question – When was this nation of ours at its healthiest? The answer is during the Second World War. "Dig for Victory" was the slogan on all the posters. I was brought up on a council estate but in those days we all had large gardens and most people used their gardens for keeping chickens, unheard of today, growing vegetables without the use of pesticides and sprays. Organic food was the order of the day. Derris dust, Jeyes fluid and soot from the chimney were the "pesticides" used to great effect. Food tasted like real food, no plasticised foods were available, no sugar, rationing at its height and yet even with the stress of war the nation remained slimmer and healthier.

Look what has happened now in the year 2010. Obesity has tripled in thirty years, diabetes is rampant, and heart conditions are the order of the day, high blood pressure, liver complaints, kidney transplants, and cancer at an all time high. The cost to the NHS is astronomical. We need to invest in our schoolchildren, educate them about diet and the consequences of wrong food intake. The estimate for the subsidisation of schoolchildren in Italy is £1700 per child per annum. What is it in this country? I suggest it is not a fraction of this figure.

In essence what I am trying to get over to you is this – I wrote my first book outlining these problems in 1984. What has changed? I would suggest to you not a lot. It is more important than ever with modern food production that we eat healthy food and create healthy bodies. I mentioned obesity earlier and the problems it can bring are multi-factorial. Here is just one example.

Dear Mr Davies,
My name is Cantie and I am 13 years old. All my life, or at least as far back as I can remember, I have had a constant headache, which often got worse and became a migraine. I was both fat and tall which made me feel clumsy and useless. I was always the biggest in my class, not just the tallest but the fattest too. I was bullied all the time about my weight and so by the time I went to public school I had no confidence left.

I found as I got older, the more I wanted to sleep. In fact life seemed very tiring and so I just slept. I played truant from games at school because I hated having to go outside with my skirt straining and my thighs flopping about, it was awful. I also missed a lot of school because I was forever ill with flu or migraine or a throat infection. To make matters worse I was dyslexic and had a memory like a sieve. I tried every sort of diet there was – or nearly – but nothing worked. I never lost a pound. In the summer term I began to get very bad stomach pains which occurred every time I ate anything. Therefore, I missed a lot of school and came bottom in every one of my exams. I had been to our local doctor several times about my pains, but I was pressed and prodded and told I was growing too fast.

One day a friend suggested that I might be allergic to certain foods and told us about Mr Davies. We went to see him and what a difference! He actually believed me about my pains and headaches; he could almost tell what I was going to say before I said it! I was taken off all dairy products, white flour, coffee, chocolate, citric acid and onions. At first the diet was hard to stick to and I had longings for chocolate and cakes, but it soon became a way of life.

I have been on the diet now for six months and so far I have lost one and a half stone and I feel great. I enjoy being outside and I would rather run than walk! My hair has stopped being lank and greasy and is now shiny and wavy. I no longer have stomach pains or headaches, and I don't feel all blocked up with sinus trouble and my eczemas has cleared up completely. I enjoy sport and I don't find work half as difficult as before. I am also much fitter and happier.

Although the diet can be an awful bore, when I do eat something I am not allowed I realise how ill I used to feel! I steer clear of sweet and cake shops but even when I do have to go in I know that the result is certainly worth it all. Mr Davies has changed my life.

Love

Cantie

I hope as you read the above letter that it awakens in you the realisation that what she is actually saying all those years ago is precisely what we are dealing with today. **Obesity. Depression. Bullying. Headaches. Fatigue and skin problems.** Does that sound like your child, or one that you know? The plain truth is that they do not need to be like it, or put up with it. Help can be found and if you need help go to my website www.gwynne-davies.com or www. gwynne.h.davies.com and look up trained Clinical Ecologists who have been trained by me. It is bad enough that Cantie had to suffer even one of those symptoms let alone a host of them. **You do not have to live with it!**

The following letter also points out that ill health can be quite a problem, but with tenacity and detective work on my part and dedication and application on yours an awful lot can be achieved. So do not give up at the first hurdle but persevere and get it right.

Halesowen
W.Midlands
Dear Mr Davies,
It has been 18 months since my first appointment with you and I would finally like to say a very big "thank you" for all your professionalism, dedication and true devotion in all your efforts with me as a patient. It must also be disheartening for you when you have expected me to improve and then I relapse for no apparent reason.

Today I feel such a sense of achievement that nothing else compares with it. My parents are truly delighted but have promised to keep an eye on their "goodies cupboard" – just in case.

I have not been happier emotionally for a long time, and now my financial problems seem to be sorting themselves out, and with my health near enough back to normal it is time to thank the ones that have helped me. You are a very caring special man who is a credit to the profession – you and your wife's dedication shows in the way you have cared for me.

I have had 21 years of hospitals, antibiotics, steroids etc; and two years later I am fitter, healthier and happier – I can't believe it is really me. I feel I have a new beginning at last and I just don't want anyone to spoil it or put me back. I would like you to know that I feel lucky to have heard of you and been treated by you.

Thank you so much. With all the respect you deserve.
Lots of Love. Debbie

This was a case where the immune system had been compromised for so long that a lot of patience and cooperation on both sides led to a successful outcome. I realise the letter is rather effusive but I have included it in the hope that you will see that application and persistence can pay off – **YOU CAN IMPROVE YOUR HEALTH!**

Chapter 3

Hyperactivity

"The time to deal with disease is one, two, ten, twenty or fifty years before it appears. But to do this on a large scale we shall have to get rid of medical science first: Because by inoculations, immunisations, radium, surgery, X-Rays, innumerable poisonous drugs, and incessant cancer, tuberculosis, germ and disease propaganda, it is disseminating and broadcasting disease, preventing recovery and proffering (at a price) an illusory would- be alternative repentance from living and obedience to the laws or conditions that govern well being. There will be fervent opposition, because as soon as the people wake up to the (still partly unconscious) fraud of medical science, eighty per cent of its "services" will not be required". This was written by Dr Ulric Williams.MB.CHB. The original Radio Doctor – Democracy NZ. 1947.

I wonder what your reaction will be when you read that statement. Having been through a horrendous war living just outside London and joining the Fleet Air Arm in 1947 I had lost touch with reality, and certainly was not aware that an opinion like that could be broadcast, and how much reaction was there. Now, 63 years later we are still facing similar pressures from the Great Pharma!! If anything it is worse. Even Governments fall prey to the propaganda and fear element they portray. The various flu epidemics, including the latest swine flu epidemic are a classic example. All the millions that were spent stocking up for the pandemic that did not happen, yet again, has to be recouped and who is going to be bludgeoned in to buying that.

Now on to hyperactivity, and what a controversial subject this is. It raises great passion because children are involved. Whether one accepts that food could be a contributory factor or not, any practitioner should at least consider the possibility of food or colourings, additives and preservatives creating a metabolic disturbance. That comment was made in 1984 in my first book, here we are twenty six years later and the same applies. In fact it is possibly more pertinent than ever.

In the last few years articles have appeared in the national press almost on a weekly basis. Following are a few classic examples: - *"Additives leave children allergic to real food. Children are consuming so many additives that their systems cannot cope with natural whole foods such as milk, eggs, flour and nuts. Almost half the population – 45% are now reporting some form of food intolerance, up from 10% twenty years ago". Another headline by James Chapman – Science Correspondent – "345,000 children are hit by behavioural disorder. Children are suffering an epidemic of behavioural problems with up to one in twenty now seriously affected, figures suggest., Such is the scale of the problem that hundreds of thousands of youngsters are being prescribed a drug known as the 'chemical cosh' because of its ability to counter hyperactivity. Two years ago the Governments watchdog ruled that Ritalin should be given to many more children with behavioural problems despite parents complaints that it turned their sons and daughters into 'zombies'. The cost to the NHS is £3.85 million a year."*

Ritalin – Methylphenidate Hydrochloride. The manufacturers in the USA are CIBA. These are the warnings they publish – "this drug should never be given to children under the age of six". "Safety and efficacy of Ritalin in long term use has never been established. Suppression of growth and weight gain has been reported with long term use". Look up Ritalin on the internet and you will find it is classed as an amphetamine likened to cocaine and incredibly addictive. There is a wonderful book by William J.Crook M.D. which I will list in the books to read section. This is beautifully illustrated and I recommend you to read it.

I am a father, grandfather and great grandfather. I care

passionately about children and their health and to give them a chance to lead a normal life. I have appeared on radio and television advising parents to try the alternative route and not allow their children to take Ritalin. It is mind numbing – it is zombie making. It does have side effects and it is not at all easy to withdraw from it. It should be supervised. I have treated hundreds of children with hyperactivity/hyperkinesis/attention deficit syndrome, and, once they have been shown what happens when tested and are on the wrong foods etc; they are the ones that set the standard; they know what happens and they do not like it. Let me quote you the following please.

Wisconsin Miracle Proves Diet Affects Behaviour

A quiet revolution has begun in Appleton, Wisconsin, USA. It started at the Central Alternative High School. The children now behave. The hallways aren't frantic. Even the teachers are happy.

The school used to be out of control. Kids packed weapons. Discipline problems swamped the principal's office. But not since 1997.

In 1997, a private group called Natural Ovens of Manitowoc, Wisconsin, underwrote a Wellness and Nutrition Programme at the school. A natural bakery was founded by Paul Stitt, a food biochemist, and Barbara Stitt who has a PhD in nutrition. Natural Ovens contributed over US$100,000 for the construction of a kitchen, provided two cooks and paid excess food bills at the high school. Teachers as well as students committed themselves to the program and, before implementing it, the staff removed all soda and junk food vending machines from the buildings.

The menu consisted of fresh fruit and vegetables, whole grain breads, homemade soups and stews and entrees. One important item that is available to students and teachers each day is the "energy drink" consisting of fruit juice, whole fruit and ground flax 'energy mix'. The flax contains Omega 3 fatty acids that are known to provide important nutrients for brain functioning.

The behaviour, stamina, attitude and health of the students and staff have improved for the better. Staff members are reporting improved attention, improvement in attendance and co-operation among students and willing to tackle complex concepts. Students report that they are also incorporating better nutrients outside school. Grades are up, truancy is no longer a problem, arguments are rare and teachers able to spend their time teaching.

The program, now in its fourth year, has been an overwhelming success and is being adopted in other Wisconsin schools. Principal LuAnn Coenen, who files annual reports with the State of Wisconsin, has turned in some staggering figures since 1997. Drop outs? Students expelled? Students discovered to be using drugs? Carrying weapons? Committing suicide? Every category has come up zero every year.

Sources: Pfeiffer Pfacts, Illinois, USA, Summer 2002. http://www.hripticorg/The Moore report.http://www.moore foundation.com.

There really is not a lot I can add to that. The evidence is there for all to see. However, let us bring the conclusion of this report nearer to home. I would like to include a story that was published in the National Association of Nursery Care by a nursing sister who brought her daughter Holly to see me.

Sharing the Caring by Jenny Davis

How many times have we heard a mother say 'I can't think what's got into him today.' But I wonder how many of you realise the truth that lies behind those few words. I don't doubt that when you have finished reading this article you will look at that statement, the children and their diet in a very different light.

Imagine my joy in finding myself pregnant. After a good pregnancy and a short labour my little Holly was born. She was beautiful, perfect, I cried.

I had already decided that I was going to breast feed and all went well; she fed well and I enjoyed it. Unfortunately the Nursing Home insisted that you were not disturbed at night and so baby was given a bottle. Those bottles were the beginning of our problems. By the fourth day Holly already had a reputation with the night staff as being difficult. When we came home things improved a little as she had very few complement feeds. Those of you who have breast fed will know the pressure that is put on you by well meaning people that if baby cries, it's because she's hungry and you haven't got enough milk, so top her up. Not knowing anything better I did so and things got worse. By four months I gave up convinced I was a failure. (My second baby may I point out, I fed for nine months and didn't listen to anyone).

Holly was put on the bottle and things got worse. I was like a zombie. She slept for about an hour during the day and four at night, interrupted with feeds and crying. My husband was marvellous and took a lot of the load, but I still felt a wreck. We all went to the doctor, who viewed us with mild amusement and prescribed Phenergan for Holly, which was supposed to knock her out. It did exactly the opposite – we now know that this was due to the colouring in the medicine. By 10 months she was walking, talking a little, she did not sleep at all during the day and was constantly moaning. The nights were awful – I was in and out of bed all night. As a matter of interest not all hyperkinetic children have a sleep problem.

I tried the doctor again and he referred us to a consultant paediatrician whose only statement was "that Holly was a dynamic baby and why should she sleep?" We left with me in tears. I thought 'damn them all – I will get through this alone'.

By the time Holly was 14 months, I was feeling really down, I couldn't seem to cope with the house, and our marriage was put under tremendous strain. There never seemed to be a moment together; our love life was hopeless with Holly always crying or when she was older, standing beside the bed; you never knew when she would walk in on you. I became neurotic about noise when she was asleep, which floorboards made a noise, never pulled the flush – even disconnected the door bell. I felt I needed an outlet, so with a friend, we started a Pram and Toddlers Group. I enjoyed it very much, but it did very little for Holly – she ran around like a whirlwind.

I have always thought that an only child was wrong – it didn't seem fair – but at the time the thought of another baby made me feel ill. When Holly was three we decided to take the plunge and try for another, hoping that a baby would help us all, she loved everyone else's baby so much. When we told her we were going to have a baby she was thrilled, however, when he arrived the story changed. She was so jealous I could not believe it. I couldn't change him without Holly going and doing something naughty. Every time I started to feed she would want something and it was always, "Its not fair, you always have Peter". Our friend suggested I give up breast feeding, but I didn't see why Peter should be deprived. Life was hell and I hated her for all the unhappiness she brought me, all the things I couldn't do, places we wouldn't dare go. I could feel the atmosphere when we went to friends – only one or two gave me total support and would even invite me when Holly was really awful. I would never want to relive those first two months with the new baby again.

I was at breaking point – something had to be done. The doctor had given me ***Valium*** *for her to try and get some peace but it made her wild, she lay on the hall floor and screamed "DON'T TOUCH ME!" I was getting to the point where I was afraid to smack Holly or even get cross in case I couldn't stop. On one occasion I shut her in her room and rang my husband to come home. I was so afraid that if she went on I would really hurt her.###*

A friend put forward a suggestion. She had been to a private clinic to be tested for food allergies to try and help her with her depression. She had been helped so much that she thought it may be worth taking Holly to see if she was allergic to any foods. We went as a family TO THE Clinic to meet Mr Davies. To my amazement he was not at all surprised at our story or at Holly's behaviour. I told him how much worse her behaviour became after she had been to a birthday party.

He was very sweet with Holly and asked her to sit on his couch. He said he was going to see if different foods made her arm strong or wobbly. He put a tiny bit of each different food under her tongue and then with her right elbow tucked tightly in to her side, he gently pushed her hand towards her chest and asked her to resist if she could. The first test was for tea and Holly was able to resist his pressure thus showing she was not allergic. Then came coffee, Mr Davies asked Holly to resist but as he applied the pressure and she tried to resist, her arm went wobbly. She turned to me and the expression of fear and wonderment on her face as to why she had no strength, told me this was no fix.

With a sip of water between each test, Mr Davies continued. At the end I was bemused, she had shown she was allergic to coffee, chocolate, citrus, white flour, white sugar, cow's milk products, cheese, colouring and preservatives, including flavourings, peas and bananas came under the colourings as they produce their own natural colourings. What was I going to feed her on? Mr Davies warned us that she may well suffer from withdrawal symptoms for the first week. In fact things went really well. I decided we would all go on Holly's diet. I emptied my cupboards of any foods she could not have and gave it all away. I was determined this had to be the answer.

The first week was like an answer to a prayer. Within two days she began to sleep thirteen or fourteen hours a night and I would find her asleep on the floor in the lounge. This excess of sleep lasted about five days, then as now, she sleeps for about ten hours. The jealousy eased towards the baby and her general attitude to everyone changed. I began to enjoy seeing her first thing in the morning – a feeling I had not experienced for a long time. I also had to learn to love her.

The diet was a little tricky until I had worked out some substitutes. We have 100% whole wheat flour bread and 85% for cakes and pastry. I make my own baking powder from rice flour, bi-carbonate of soda and cream of tartar. We have pure cane sugar instead of white, goat milk instead of cow, animal rennet free cheese and Mazola oil instead of margarine for cooking. I have become a compulsive label reader and if it doesn't say what's in it, I don't buy it.

Everything was going really well, people who knew Holly remarked on the change, but we were not out of the woods yet. After several weeks of what seemed like heaven, Holly began to get difficult at bedtime and sometimes during the day. Then one day it clicked as she came and told for the third time that morning that she had cleaned her teeth. I rushed upstairs and looked at the toothpaste tube. It was nearly empty. I couldn't believe it – she was eating the toothpaste! It never occurred to me that the stripe in the new tube would have any effect on her, but she felt it, and began to crave it. I changed the toothpaste and everything returned to normal.

After something like twelve months of good days and nights we begun to have problems .Her teacher also noticed the change and wondered if it was the excitement of the approaching Christmas Nativity play, but I could see all the old signs returning as well. Constant uncontrolled laughter, silly faces, wild eyes and the old faithful bad nights and the constant movement. I rang Mr Davies and he said "I think we had better have a retest".

On arriving at West Highlands, Mr Davies greeted Holly like an old friend, smiled at me and said "Yes, I can see it". I told him an average day's menu and he started the tests. He hadn't gone far when goat milk showed as an allergy. (Lactose intolerance – Author). Both of us were surprised – where do we go from here? Soya milk is the answer. She was also allergic this time to the white of egg but this didn't pose too much of a problem as I just gave her two yolks So, we plod on again once more with a pleasant child. However, we have taken care not to give Holly any food drink in excess as it is possible for her to build an allergy to it. An interesting point I think, is that food allergies seem to run in families. If there is a child with a behaviour problem – look at the family; does anyone have asthma, eczema, migraine, hay fever, depression, ear infections or even a skin or intestinal problem? If they do, it is quite possible that their problem and the child's behaviour could be due to food allergies although not in all cases.

I have now started a local group for mothers of children who have been tested by Mr Davies. Not all the children are first babies or only children. We give support and swap ideas for recipes. I hope that that some of you, having read this article, will be able to see that something could be done to help a child, or perhaps a family you know. Let there be a happy end to the sad story of hyperkinetic children.

Jenny Davis.

I know parents must get desperate in situations like this, but for the life of me I cannot imagine what a doctor was doing giving a small child Valium. Read up the side effects!

When this was written soya milk was the only alternative. Now there is rice milk, almond milk, oat milk and organic soya milk.

Your last paragraph is a wonderful sentiment Jenny; I wish it were to be true, but sad to say that the situation, six years since my last publication has not changed. I have said many times in my retirement that I would love to go in to schools and talk not only to the children but the parents and teachers as well. I hope that this book will awaken parents with "difficult" children to the fact that they do not need to suffer. I have trained practitioners in the field and they are on my web site www.gwynnedavies.com.

Are you a teacher? Perhaps you recognise that disruptive child in your class, or maybe even more than one. They cannot sit still, fidgeting all the time, twiddling with their pencil, twisting their hair through their fingers all the time, is slow to respond and finds it difficult to concentrate. You could do this child a great service. You could suggest to the parents that hyperkinesis is not unusual; it carries no stigma, but is recognised in many cases as being related to allergy. With your guidance and understanding of the problem the parents will no doubt seek help, and another child destined for the scrap heap will be able to lead a normal life.

November 2010 – Headline in national newspaper. **1 IN 4 BOYS LABELLED WITH SPECIAL NEEDS.** It states that this is caused by behavioural and emotional problems. How much of this is allergy – food sensitivity – vaccination? When the authorities insist on vaccinating with Vitamin K and HIB in the first few weeks it is not surprising when one knows the contents of these vaccines.

The story of Holly gives you some idea of how bad it can be, but I would ask you to bear with me while I relate the most serious case I have ever had, and that runs in to many hundreds. This serious case was when I was practising in Northern Germany.

Bernt was an eight year old boy who from birth had been difficult, never sleeping properly, crying a lot, being restless and bad tempered to the point of uncontrollable rages where everything within reach was thrown. In short, an impossible child. The parents approached their general practitioner who prescribed a 'drug' to quieten him down. This worked initially to ease the situation but was not the answer. The next step was a psychologist and further 'drugs' were used, year after year but no relief was obtained. Bernt continued to be a 'difficult child'. Note please that I have never found that 'drugs' had any other effect on children than a deleterious one. He was eight years of age for goodness sake!

For those of you who have to deal with autism the following will ring a few bells. Bernt never asked for or gave affection to his parents. If they tried to give him a hug he shrugged them off with a curse. In the end his behaviour was so intolerable that they firmly believed he was possessed of the devil. They agreed to Bernt being admitted to a specialised psychiatric unit in

Southern Germany. Like Holly's parents the strain was so bad that they were on the point of divorce.

Five days prior to his committal his Auntie who was a nursing sister in Neumunster hospital, and a patient of mine, asked if I thought it was worth while bringing Bernt to me as a last resort. How often have I heard that statement – the last resort? I naturally informed the Aunt that at that stage anything was worth a try. She rang the parents straight away and they set off from Berlin on a five hour drive to my practice in North Germany.

They brought the 'horror' in to my clinic, struggling and cursing under his breath, no way was he going to co-operate. Within minutes he was around the room picking things up and displacing them, I asked the parents to sit down and not take any notice of him. I tried to get them to understand my hypothesis that there is no such thing as a 'bad' child under the age of twelve. There was always a reason - a "trigger". He was not possessed by the devil or evil spirits but was being over activated by one or more allergens to food or substances.

Naturally they looked at me with total disbelief, how could a few foods create such a destructive reaction? I then explained that I had seen many children nearly as bad as their son, and they had responded well and were now "normal" children and I saw no reason why their son should not be the same. Slowly I saw a change in the parent's attitude and a glimmer of interest from Bernt, especially when I said that I was going to see how strong his arm was. He could not resist that challenge. He agreed to be tested and I found him hypersensitive to five foods and colourings. They were almost identical to those found in Holly. I warned the parents that we may not see any improvement for days, and could even get worse. Our time was terribly limited. At least Bernt agreed to co-operate as he had no wish to leave home and go to a "special school".

Exactly five days later I received a phone call from the mother.

For the first time in his life he had gone in to his parents' bedroom, sat on the edge of the bed, put his arm round his mother's neck and said, "Mein liebe Mutti, Ich liebe dich" – my dear mother I love you. The very first signs of affection and just in the nick of time – we had a breakthrough. The small miracle we had prayed for had happened. (I still get a lump in my throat when I relate that story). How the parents must have felt beggars belief. It was not all plain sailing of course; Bernt still had his problems if he ingested toxic substances.

On one occasion he sneaked off to his bedroom not aware that his mother was watching him through a crack in the door. He started revolving on the spot, faster and faster until he was very red in the face and panting. He stamped his foot, cursed under his breath and said "why can't I get angry and upset, it used to work before? I must have some cake". So, you see he was well aware that having the wrong food etc could trigger a response. I am delighted to say that he did not eat the cake and he was leading a perfectly normal life last time I heard from them. The lovely thing is that they now have a son who shows affection and love for his parents and the new arrival in the family.

It will mean that once the problems for the child are resolved the problems for the parents begin. Shopping initially will be far from easy and certainly will be time consuming. But like riding a bike or driving a car, once you get the hang of it life will be much easier and shopping much quicker. You will need to read labels avidly, and believe me manufacturers do not make life easy for you. The print is usually microscopic and the technical jargon used on occasions is only decipherable by reference. I would suggest very strongly that you obtain the booklet Find Out - £5 - from Foresight, 178 Hawthorn Road, Aldwick, Bognor Regis, West Sussex. PO21 2UY. This booklet is beautifully presented in traffic light sequence, so, very easy to decipher. Red for danger, amber for caution, green for go.

It will be of great advantage if the whole family go the same way of eating; I only refer to it as a diet for speed of recognition. If the whole family adopt the new way of eating it avoids any petty jealousies arising with siblings and parents. The easiest way is to avoid all additives, colourings and flavourings. Keep to the whole foods, fresh vegetables, fresh fruits (in season), and buy organic whenever possible. If you have the ground, why not try growing your own? The food tastes better and is cheaper by far. If you cannot grow your own then try one of the organisations in the Appendix. In most towns these days there are box schemes for the delivery of organic or home grown foods. If you doubt my word as to how good they are, take a carrot from the supermarket and one from local organic supplier, you will not believe the difference in taste and texture.

Chapter 4

Migraine and Neurological Conditions

The official version

A common and distressing kind of headache, with no evident cause.

Attacks last a few hours.(1) They may be frequent but some people have only one or two typical attacks in a lifetime. (2) Warning symptoms such as a sense of flickering before the eyes are common: during the attack the patient cannot stand bright light. Most patients feel nauseated during or after the attack and some actually vomit. The classic accounts of migraine describe the headaches as being one sided. (3) This is quite common but by no means the rule.

The site of the trouble seems to be the arteries inside and outside the skull, but the nature and the cause of migraine are still unknown. (4) It has no lasting effects (5) and the attacks become less frequent with time.(6). Over activity of a substance such as histamine and serotonin, that affects the relaxation and contraction of the arteries, is the likeliest explanation of migraine (7). One must then account for the over activity. (8). Emotional upset, perhaps acting through such substances plays some part but is not the main factor. (9).

Many different kinds of treatment work in particular cases, suggesting that migraine might have many causes. (10). When anti-histamine drugs work, for example, this is a strong hint that the attacks may be allergic. (11). Drugs derived from ergot are perhaps more often effective than any others, but until the causes are better understood the treatment of migraine will remain a matter of trial and error. (12).

The figures in brackets are points I would like to address,

expand upon or take issue with.

I would certainly agree that it is a most distressing condition, and if you have not suffered with migraine, I doubt you will have any conception of the intensity of the pain. I have watched a dear friend of mine for years, suffering the agonies of migraine for as much as three days at a time. He died quite young with a cerebral embolism. I still feel sadness to this day that I did not have the knowledge then that I have today. I feel sure I could have saved him.

With no evident cause. In all my years in practice and treating many hundreds of migraine sufferers, if I looked for the cause – I found it! In most cases it was "triggered" by a sensitivity to certain foods, in some cases it needed a cervical spine osteopathic manipulation, and in the case of many women patients it needed a hormonal adjustment.(1).

Remember the dear old pancreas? The instigatory endochrine/ excocrine organ of the body. Our central computer! It controls our brain function and our central nervous system by producing noradrenaline and norepinephrine, serotonin and glutathione, producing symptoms such as temporal lobe epilepsy, schizophrenia(bi-polar), migraine, panic attacks and chronic anxiety, in other words conditions that are exacerbated by tension or stress.

Try and picture what I was describing earlier about the mast cells. Remember we are compartmentalised like a ship. So we are talking about the head. Because of a pancreatic malfunction (allergy) antibodies are being produced and attaching themselves to the mast cells, the adrenal glands are under stress and atrophying (shrinking). Therefore the amount of adrenaline, cortisone and histamine being produced is lessened, at identically the same time the mast cells become saturated, the adrenalin gland exhausted and the mast cells shrug off the antibodies and they flood in to the brain compartment – outcome – migraine.

(2) The attacks last a few hours. I would hotly dispute this as

I have had many patients with severe migraine that last for as long as three to five days. It goes without saying that can leave the patient "wiped out" for days afterwards. (3) The headaches are one sided. Not in my experience. It does happen but in most cases of severe migraine the skull feels as though it is being torn apart(4) the cause and nature of migraine unknown. I agree that it can be puzzling in some cases, but in every case I dealt with there was a reason. (5) It has no lasting effect. I wonder what is meant by that. Every single patient without fail reported that the migraine left them totally exhausted for days afterwards.

(6) The attacks diminish in time. Sorry, I found exactly the opposite. The migraine started by appearing once or twice a year, then to once a month, then every few weeks, and in some cases as much as once a week. (7) the production of serotonin and histamine. I go along with that, the pancreatic malfunction determines that this takes place and one of the classics is the ingestion of strawberries which have a high content of histamine. So be warned!! (8) A matter of trial and error. I have already said that in my experience this was never the case.

Some years ago now I carried out 27 TV Broadcasts on health matters with Jenny Smedley. One of the ladies that came on the programme called Carol had followed the classic pattern for 32 years – she was 38 years of age, she had at least one severe migraine a week. It affected her life in every way; she had difficulty holding down a job as she was continually off sick. Her love life was affected; in fact she was functioning at a very low level most of the time. We tested her and removed dairy products, because she was manifesting other symptoms from the age of six, then we removed the 4C's – coffee, cheese, citrus and chocolate. Because of the possibility of peripheral reactions we also removed temporarily tomato and hazelnuts.

As predicted she had a few really bad days but then her head cleared and she was feeling good until three days before her menses – migraine! A hormonal involvement so we addressed this by introducing Agnus Castus and Phytoestrol. I am delighted to report that providing she keeps to the restrictive way of eating she is fine. She has since taken a top executive job in Cornwall.

I hope you will bear with me including a few letters from patients but I do feel that if you can read what other people are saying it will encourage you to go ahead and do something about it.

Knutsford
Cheshire
Dear Mr Davies,
It is now over six months since I saw you at the beginning of June. I thought you may like some indication of my progress as, in many cases, I assume you do not get any 'feed back'. At the time of my visit I had suffered with serious migraines for over twenty years. I was losing time off work at the rate of about 2/3 days a month. My family life was seriously affected – week ends particularly and holidays where father had to stay in a darkened room for the first few days away!

Edmund and Hazel Preston suggested I see you and to say I was very sceptical would be understating the position, but, as my wife and partners said, what had I to lose. You made three predictions after you had tested me. Because of the strength of the test doses I would have an attack before I got as far as Birmingham, that when I started your diet I would have the worst attack that I had ever experienced and thirdly, that if I stuck to the diet I would have no more migraines.

All this turned out to be true. The attack on the way home cleared up later that night, the later attack was indeed the worst ever and the visual effects took several weeks to clear up. I have tried to experiment with the diet to see if I can vary it – I can, but not by very much. Due to such 'experiments' I have lost 2 days from the office in 6 months.

My partners and my family are delighted. My wife now realises what it is like to live with a normal human being. Until now I have never been migraine free throughout our marriage. She has proved very helpful in obtaining the foods allowed on the diet and she is of the view the family's diet has improved as a result .I owe you a large debt of gratitude. Long may your good work continue. Best wishes

Yours sincerely

H.L.(Male)

Highclere

Newbury

Berks

Dear Mr Davies,

It is now just over two months since I came to see you, since when I have followed the diet rigidly which you prescribed.

There have been many days, or occasions, when previously I would have had a migraine attack, but since the one which I had (as you foretold) at the very beginning) there hasn't been one. The frequent feeling of slight sickness has gone, and I have never felt fitter.

To say that I am grateful is an understatement! It has made all the difference to my enjoyment of life. To be able to eat vegetarian cheese, and drink Kalibu milk, reduces the sense of deprivation quite considerably. So, thank you very much indeed. I hope that I never have to trouble you again.

Yours sincerely. W.P.S. (Male)

I have deliberately included letters from men, for the simple reason that women were the predominant patients and I could include many letters from them. You will note that I made three predictions. I would never have been able to do such a thing without the experience of many years and hundreds of migraine patients. With severe migraine cases it was predictable what would happen in every case. The pattern never changed. Within

12-14 hours of withdrawing the "trigger" foods the reactions would begin. Invariably the migraine was the worst ever encountered, and in many cases included vomiting. If you reach the stage of what I call 'dry retching' then either ring the doctor yourself or get a partner or family member to do it for you. Explain that you have been to see me and what is happening. He will come and give you an injection of Pethidine or Stemetil or both. This will allow things to calm down and allow you to recover. But I do stress again – **call your doctor!**

Once you have passed through this withdrawal phase which can be quite traumatic, it is almost certain you will never have another migraine. The inevitable question is bound to be raised at some time, "when can I re-introduce the foods I am allergic to". Once you have been without migraine for three months it is worthwhile, (but not always), to introduce a small cup of coffee, the odd square of chocolate but never on the same day or in close proximity. It is worth trying tomato again and hazelnut, but, the one thing you will have to watch very carefully is citrus. It can be lethal.

I treated one lady patient who had suffered with severe migraines for years and she went through all the expected trauma of withdrawal, and had been well for several months. She was invited out to close friends for dinner, she naturally informed her hostess of her "trigger" foods and was assured that there would be nothing problematic in the meal. The starter and main course were fine- then came the dessert. It was based on apple but when she started to eat it she noticed that her tongue tingled and she did not feel quite right. When they removed from the dining room she approached the hostess and told her what had happened, she was assured immediately that there was nothing wrong – then her face went white and she told my patient that she had soaked the apples in lemon juice to prevent them going brown. My patient excused herself and left the party immediately, hurriedly making her apologies, and drove the twenty miles home, parked the car, and all she remembers is putting the key in the door. Her husband heard this and waited and when she did not appear went to the front door and found his wife collapsed on the doorstep.

Once indoors the husband rang me and I advised him to make up a teaspoon of bicarbonate of soda and mix with warm water. Lift her head and slowly drip this solution under her tongue and she recovered quite quickly. Should you be aware that you have ingested something that is wrong you can do the same and save a lot of discomfort. However, it is a first aid remedy only and not be used frequently. I know this was an extreme case but it does sometimes happen. Great care must be taken at all times.

If you cheat, you cheat only one person - yourself!!

When migraine is mentioned one naturally thinks of a severe headache. This is not always the case. I have had hundreds of patients suffering with severe pains in the stomach and gut, but, no headache at all or only of minor importance to them. The overriding symptoms were the gut pains, sometimes to the point of doubling them up – bowel cramps? They are very painful too, like a migraine. These symptoms I term – gut migraine! Eliminate the foods I have mentioned previously and the pains will inevitably dissipate very quickly.

The next statement I make is not scientifically proven, and I would like to make that absolutely clear. It is my hypothesis, but based on what I have observed over the years in association with migraine headaches. It is my belief that the continual barrage of adverse symptoms attacking the brain and causing such distressing results can lead to stroke or ischaemic attacks. If any organ is attacked repeatedly there is going to be a response of some kind. Are neurological conditions of any kind the responsibility of the same toxins that create migraine? Alzheimers, dyslexia, dementia, multiple sclerosis, depression, many years ago the medical opinion was that the blood/brain barrier could not be crossed. It is now proven beyond doubt that it can be breached. So, I wonder, will my hypothesis become fact? I really do not see why not.

Multiple Sclerosis

The following is a letter received two days ago followed by quoting a male case in Bristol.

Dear Mr Davies

About 21 years ago I was diagnosed with Multiple Sclerosis. The specialist said it was Progressive M.S. with no known cure. I asked what I could do and was told 'I wouldn't have hot baths if I were you'. I felt there was no help and I could only get worse. I was very frightened and there did not seem anyone I could turn to.

After reading a book on "How to manage M.S."I had read in three separate paragraphs that smoking, too much fat and sugar were all bad for you. I gave up all three and lost 3 stone in 3 months! I was losing weight at 2lbs a week and one of my daughters actually said to me one day 'be careful in the shower Mum, you might go down the plug hole'.

My brother told me about one of his salesmen who worked for him in his caravan sales business who had been helped with his crippling arthritis by Gwynne.H.Davies in Taunton. He had improved so much that he moved to France and opened a Hotel. My brother obtained Gwynne's number from him and suggested I gave Gwynne a ring. I did not know who else to turn to.

I rang the number and a cheerful lady answered, Mrs Davies (Rosemarie). I asked if they saw people with M.S. and she said "of course, please come along for an appointment", or words to that effect. Anyway it turned out to be the best thing I have ever done. The first consultation I had with Mr Davies, I didn't know what to expect, after talking to me for half an hour he then said "I can't cure you but I can help you".

After tears of relief he then proceeded to test me with his special method of finding my allergies. From that day I stopped losing weight and over the next months, after removing all the toxins and allergies from my diet (not very easy at first), I started regaining my weight at a rate of 1lb a week and started to improve.

Over the last 19 years at least I have not had a headache and I don't perspire. I have so much energy most days that I get up at 7am and rarely go to bed before 11pm. I am active throughout the day, so much so that I keep getting told to sit down and rest, but, I don't sit down for long!

I am improving all the time, slowly but surely. Sadly the only thing I won't get back is my balance but I can live with that. I do also get tired in hot weather, but I don't suffer with fatigue which is normal with M.S.

The good thing that has come from having M.S. is meeting Gwynne Davies and his lovely wife Rosemarie. Also his then secretary Anne Reilly who was extremely helpful. I can not them enough, they have always been there for me and always had time to listen to me and advise me. They are also helping my daughter Anna and granddaughter Jenna. We are very grateful and feel very privileged. Best of all I was given hope.

I thank you so much Mr Davies. YOU'RE THE BEST!

Mrs A.McEwan (Anita)

Weston-Super-Mare.

Thank you Anita, not for your very kind comments about us both but the message I hope it gives **HOPE AND RELIEF** to the many hundreds of M.S sufferers out there. If you know of anyone or are treating someone with the condition tell them to read this book. My only comment about the letter is that Anita has not had her amalgam fillings removed, and I feel strongly as do many of my colleagues, Dr Patrick Kingsley in particular, that until they are removed the balance cannot be restored.

The other case that springs to mind, and there are many, is

John from Bristol. He had been in a wheelchair for 17 years and as well as M.S. had scoliosis of the spine. I know he will not mind me saying that he was in a bad way, unable to speak clearly, movement of limbs very restricted. Within months this man was able to practise his first love and trade, woodwork by making me 2 coffee tables. I am still in touch with the family so I do know how things are going to this day. So all you M.S. sufferers **DO NOT DESPAIR** – you can be helped, but most important of all **YOU CAN HELP YOURSELVES** with the right advice. I will be putting the names and addresses of people I have trained and are using my methods to this day at the back of the book.

Dyslexia

This is one condition that I was not familiar with for many years. I knew what it was, I had a gut feeling that one of my children suffered from it, but I had not had a patient with this condition. I then started reading books about dyslexia, I spoke to a friend of mine who was the Director of the British Institute for Brain Injured Children. I had been talking to him about the book by Philpott and Kalita called Brain Allergies the Psychonutrient Connection and the association between mental function and food sensitivity. He explained to me that one of the primary things they found at the Institute for brain injured children was that, on questioning, the parents offered the information that their child had never crawled. The first signs of the essential cross patterning were not there. The children either skated across the floor on their bottoms, or their potty, or stood straight up and tottered about walking. So, the very first mental stimulus to the left and right sides of the brain were not "triggered".

This made me think of the numerous times I had heard migraine patients say their headaches were mainly left or right sided. The other thing they found difficult was not being able to watch television or read because of visual disturbance. I then recalled reading somewhere about Human Ecology and

Balancing Sciences (HEBS), the kinesiological testing of muscle/nerve/brain reflexes. Somewhere along the line I remembered associating this with something I had read in a book about dyslexia. It sounded rather complicated and far fetched but nothing should be dismissed out of hand until proved one way or another.

Not long after recalling this a young lad of twelve was brought to see me. He was the son of a very well known MP and had been to see specialists and psychiatrists, but nothing seemed to help. He was underweight and undersize for his age. Even though he was at a prestigious public school, Harrow, he was bullied and third from bottom in his class. I explained to the parents how the pancreas affects not only the physical but brain function too. He was classified as dyslexic and had special tutoring at school. I suggested it would be worth while trying the Rochlitz method once the basic "triggers" were eliminated. He was keen to try and so were the parents.

On testing it was no surprise to me that he was allergic to dairy products and the 4C Syndrome. Coffee, cheese, citrus, chocolate – the same allergies as most migraine sufferers. I explained the Rochlitz Test to them. Stand with back resting against a wall – place a clock so it is easily seen – commence by counting the clock round from 12 round to 12 and reverse – at the same time humming a favourite tune – at the same time lifting the right leg and patting the left hand on the knee – replace – and raise the left leg and patting the knee with the right hand. **Cross patterning/crawling motion.** So you see three things are being carried out at the same time oral/physical/visual. It is possible that you can not get the hang of all three at once, so start with two, watching the clock round and back and humming.

This exercise should be carried out three times a day for at least three weeks, in severe cases longer. During this time of course the detoxification process is taking place. Because of the possible hereditary IgE factor his mother came to see me some months later. I asked how her son was and she told me the sequel. The parents were asked to go to Harrow and see the Headmaster – he asked them what on earth had happened to their son over the Christmas holidays, and subsequently, that had brought about an amazing transformation. He had grown an inch and a half in one term, he was so bright he had gone from third bottom in class to third top – and on seeing the psychologist was found not to be dyslexic any more. They informed the Head that they had brought their son to see me and his response was, "oh! That man again, several of our masters have been to see him". Full credit to the school the Matron had ensured that his dietary exclusions were adhered to. As I am sure you can imagine that word spread like wildfire and I was inundated with dyslexic patients. I am delighted to say that providing 'the straight and narrow' was adhered to it worked every time. But again I must stress make sure you see a trained Clinical Ecologist.

Epilepsy

What a frightening condition this can be. The petit mal where the eyes go blank and there is 'no one at home' is bad enough. But a grand mal, a full seizure is so frightening for the parent or onlooker, and certainly no fun for the patient. Although most times they are not aware of what has happened. Again I have to stress that I am hypothesising but it must do some damage to the brain cells each time. This is why the drugs used to control epilepsy are so powerful. Some people find it difficult to cope with the condition and the case long ago of the 'royal prince' who was kept away from the rest of the family because of the condition is a classic. I treated epileptic adults and children for over twenty years with much scepticism from the medical fraternity. Now I am pleased to say it is accepted that there could be a link between the fits and food sensitivity. Maybe I was before my time.

I am sure that once you have read Brain Allergies the

Psychonutrient Connection then it will all make sense. The worst case I ever saw was an eighteen year old young man from Weston-Super-Mare who was on the maximum allowable medication and was still fitting 7-17 times a day. The mother was very frightened as he was a big chap and liable to hurt her as well as himself. With such a serious case I wondered whether anything could be achieved, so I asked the mother to contact her doctor and tell him what we were attempting to do, and if he was in any doubt to read Brain Allergies.

Thankfully even when he was going through the withdrawal phase the fits did not get any worse but slowly diminished. After three weeks he was on the minimum medication and – no fits! It goes without saying that with a situation as serious as this great care must be taken controlling the dietary side of things. You cannot take chances with "trigger" foods.

I am reminded all these years later of my colleague the Director of the Institute for Brain Injured Children. He was so scathing initially and sceptical about the possible link between pancreatic malfunction and the effect on the brain. His daughter was severely damaged by the whooping cough vaccine and was about 11 or 12 when I first met her. She had constant fits every day, but thankfully the mother, a physiotherapist, was not so scathing or as sceptical as her husband, and wanted help for her daughter. So, she was brought to Taunton to see me and on testing was found to be hypersensitive to dairy products, the 4C syndrome and colourings and additives. Once we eliminated these she improved. But, she still had fits. Admittedly not as many but they were still apparent.

She contracted tonsillitis and was badly affected, did not wish to eat, and could only drink water through a straw. This lasted for several days. Something strange happened. Her behaviour and the fits improved and stopped. Voila! There must be a link between food ingestion and brain function. Even father was impressed. After five days her condition had improved enormously and her tonsillitis was getting better. As she walked past the breakfast table where the other children were eating, her hand went to her mouth, she wetted her fingers and dipped them in the sugar bowl and straight into her mouth. All done in a few seconds. She continues for another dozen or so paces and bang! – a Grand Mal! If ever any of us were in doubt there was 'the proof of the pudding'.

If you are a parent of a child with epilepsy, have a word with your doctor and suggest that you eliminate all dairy products and the 4C syndrome plus additives and colourings and where possible preservatives. I really do think there would be very few cases that would not respond. **You don't have to live with it!**

Eliminating the 4C Syndrome

Coffee

Fairly simple to eliminate as it is not usually hidden in other foods, although I have known patients react to coffee sweets. I am asked repeatedly if decaffeinated coffee is permissible. The answer is a very short and sharp NO! Coffee is coffee is coffee – OUT! There are alternative coffee substitutes available from the health shop. Bambu. Barley cup. Dandelion coffee has skimmed milk or lactose in it on occasions, choose pure dandelion root.

Chocolate

Again fairly simple to eliminate as it is obvious. If there is no allergy to dairy then Carob and Kalibu are permissible. Carob powder for cooking is very good. Where dairy is concerned or lactose intolerance beware of what were at one time safe chocolate. Green & Black's plain was always permissible but since being taken over by Kraft it now contains dairy. Divine or pure cacao is fine but strong, or Celtic dark chocolate products.

Cheese

I have found for years that the "trigger" in cheese has been the animal rennet, because of the enzymatic structure changes, these days it is difficult to find a cheese with animal rennet, just ensure it says vegetarian with a "V" symbol.

Citrus

Probably the most difficult of all the group to eliminate as it is in so many foods and drinks. Providing you are always alert and study labels carefully you should be fine. Watch for things containing Bioflavinoids they are citrus – unless stated otherwise. Avoid the following – Lemon balm tea, oranges, tangerines, lemons, limes,strawberries, tomato, citric acid, citrates, grapefruit, pineapple, rooibosch tea (temporarily).

Diet Sheet For Elimination of Toxins
Migraine and Gut Migraine

ON RISING Glass of hot water with teaspoon of honey.

BREAKFAST Corn flakes, shredded wheat, puffed rice, goat, sheep or organic soya milk. Fruit juice of choice (non citric), Darjeeling, Assam, Luaka or Green tea, Caro, Barley cup, Pionier (alternative coffee).

LUNCH Salad – organic whenever possible. Lettuce, cress, cucumber, celery, grated or shredded cabbage, beetroot, vegetarian cheese, one ryvita or slice of wheatmeal bread, beef, lamb, chicken, top fish only.(NO BOTTOM FISH plaice, dab, flounder etc;).

TEA Wheatmeal bread and honey, tea or alternative coffee.

SUPPER Avocado, Icelandic prawns, steak, lamb chops, chicken, cod, whiting, haddock, Pollock, bream, bass. Boiled or baked potato (no skin), peas, beans, lentils, cabbage, sprouts, broccoli, cauliflower, carrots.

Producing alkaline but acid in raw state

Grapefruit, orange, lemon, limes.

Alkaline in raw state but acid when cooked

Beef, lamb, chicken, pork.

Foods which can cause constipation

Coffee, cheese, salt meat, white bread, spiced foods, mixed dishes, eggs, rice, pastry, soya, condiments, pickles, tea.

Foods which can have a laxative effect

Raisins, raw cabbage, apples, wholweheat, figs, plums, prunes, pears, tomato, cauliflower, peaches, grapes, celery, grapefruit, bran, spinach, parsnips, swede, carrots.

As constipation is the scourge of society today it is worth bearing these foods in mind. This diet plan and the foods suggested are advisory and for you to chose from. Please remember the importance of drinking enough water on a daily basis. 3 litres is minimum recommended.

You will note that I have eliminated Citrus/Bioflavinoids for migraine patients.

DO NOT drink with a meal. The salivary glands produce ample water to aid mastication: drinking fluid with a meal impairs and enfeebles these glands.

NO PORK, HAM, BACON, VEAL. APPLE SKIN. APPLE JUICE. CIDER, CIDER VINEGAR.

ASPALLS OR PEAKES ORGANIC APPLE JUICE IS PERMITTED.

THIS DIET IS FOR FIVE DAYS AS A DETOX DIET – IT IS THEN LEFT TO YOUR COMMON SENSE TO EXPAND YOUR DIET WITH CAUTION.

Over the years of testing and treating neurological conditions, such as temporal lobe epilepsy, dyslexia, schizophrenia (bi-polar), manic depression, Alzheimer's and motor neurone disease, and dementia a pattern began to emerge of the foods implicated in these conditions. There were exceptions, as in the case of Alzheimer's where aluminium was a definite link to the condition. The above recommendations for migraine apply. The other link which became an essential part of the recovery programme for all but migraine, was the essential removal of mercury amalgam fillings.

This must be supervised by a clinical ecologist and an experienced dental surgeon familiar with the necessary procedures to be adopted. It still staggers me to this day in 2010 that one of the most poisonous substances known to man is placed two inches from the brain.

It is generally accepted that when a disease such as influenza reaches 400 per 100,000 or 0.4 per cent of the population, it is then considered to be of epidemic proportions. In January 1997, the British Dental Association (BDA) issued a fact file on mercury, stating "about 3% of the population are estimated to be suffering from mercury sensitivity". 3% o the UK population would represent some 1.75 million people. Despite these potentially huge figures, no action is taken on mercury toxicity and, unlike BSE and AIDS, it has attracted relatively little media attention. What is even more damning is the fact that **no public money has been allocated for research!**

However, current research suggests that mercury vapour from fillings may be one of the predominantly underlying causes of a broad spectrum of neurological conditions including Parkinson's disease. Even though I have treated these conditions over a great number of years, those that stand out in my mind, and responded most favourably were those with neurological conditions and underwent the sequential removal of mercury amalgam. It would be fair to say that if any of my patients with these conditions did not respond as hoped, and then the removal of dental mercury amalgam was the next step. It is also a matter on record that all those tested for mercury amalgam failed when tested. There are certain doctors in this country that will not take on a patient with suspected neurological condition until such times that they have had the mercury removed.

One patient in particular comes to mind, and I do not mind telling you I found the experience quite hair raising, as did my staff. The lady presented with what was diagnosed as progressive Alzheimer's disease, so on her third visit, where she was making good progress, we agreed that the next step was to test for further causatory "triggers". I did not tell her what we were going to use as I did not wish to pre-empt a response. I placed the small amount of mercury filling under her tongue, instantaneously her mouth clamped shut, her pupils dilated, she ground her teeth furiously shaking her head from side to side and emitted the most horrendous screeching. This went on for what seemed an age, but in fact was a few seconds, I tried to get my fingers in to her mouth and remove the amalgam, it was jammed shut. I reached for a syringe and pulled some Dr Bach Rescue Remedy into it and forced this between her clenched teeth, to my great relief this resolved the situation and she relaxed enough for the removal of the amalgam.

The patient had no recollection of what had happened so was not in the least perturbed. I wiped the perspiration from my brow and helped the lady from the couch. Once I was sure she was alright I told her what had happened, and she agreed to have the amalgam removed. Off she went downstairs to the office. I called the next patient and apologised for the frightening noise as she may have thought I had done something horrific. She assured me she was a doctor and I was not to be concerned. Thank goodness she was the only patient who reacted in that way, but it certainly made me ponder the long term effect on a patient with a neurological condition if a reaction could be induced that quickly.

> *"The primary cause of Alzheimer's is iatrogenic (drug induced) disease caused by chronic low level mercurial poisoning from dental amalgam fillings. Dental mercury amalgams are not stable – they undergo corrosion, and dangerous amounts of mercury vapour are daily released – this may be inhaled by the lungs and in that way enter the general blood circulation and passed into the whole body. However, far more dangerous are similarly released mercurial fumes, which, instead settle down on the mucous membranes in the upper regions of the nasal cavity, from where the mercury is transported*

directly to the brain. These pathways are either by the olfactory nerves or by the valve less cranial venous system that presents an open venous communication between the oro nasal cavity and the brain".

Patrick Stortebecker MD.PhD.

It only goes for me to say that having read numerous books, articles and my own observations, I would always advise any patient of mine to have the mercury amalgam removed by a knowledgeable dental surgeon, and only ever have the alternative filling materials which are being improved all the time. Dentists in general will tell you that these materials are less hard wearing. I was advised when I was having new false plates fitted that as it was clear composite it would not last more than five years and possibly crack before then. I am still happily wearing them and that is at least 25 years ago. Do not put yourself through a root canal filling without reading up on it. The latest book I have read on the subject is Toxic Bite by Dr Bill Kellner – Read, Credence Publications, ISBN 1-904015-00-X. He says – "everyone of us goes to the dentist. But how many of us are aware that a problem in the mouth can lead to serious, life – threatening problems in the body".

"As long ago as 1992, the German Ministry of Health declared a ban on silver mercury fillings. The German announcement contradicts the pervasive and fraudulent pronouncements by the ADA…these organisations blatantly lie when they declare silver amalgam fillings are harmless to patients…said merely to protect American dentists from legal assault by an angry public…Dr Casdorph, MD".

That is all I can say on the subject as I am not a qualified dentist. But, before you make any decision make absolutely sure you are aware of what you are undertaking and what the consequences may be. I would suggest that if you need further information contact WDDTY (What Doctor's Don't Tell You), 4

Wallace Road, London, N1 2 PG. They print a specialised booklet on mercury amalgam and dental procedures. One last thing on Alzheimer's which is vitally important – if you have a member of the family suffering with this condition or dementia please contact me on my website www.gwynnedavies.com and I will be happy to guide you through the 12 point programme for detoxification.

One other thing that comes to mind while we are on the subject of neurological conditions is toothpaste. Remember the story of Holly and her eating the toothpaste. That was the need to placate the addictive process brought about by the adrenal glands requiring something to stimulate them. Every neurological case I saw reacted to modern toothpastes and the colourings in them. I also believe that there is an element of doubt, to say the least, about fluoride and the connection between that and neurological conditions. So, I would suggest that you use one of the non- fluoride toothpastes from the Health Shop.

Fluoride

Fluoridation may reduce tooth decay in children's teeth.

(That's it. There is no other reason to fluoridate.) Note the word may – not will.

There is a mass of evidence which convinces me that fluoridation is the government and industries way of disposing of a waste product. Ethically, fluoridation is repugnant on a number of counts. It is an assumption of moral superiority. By what right do dentist's claim 'some peoples wishes can be ignored because we know what is good for you whether you like it or not". Such an attitude encourages bad medical ethics — believing it permissible to prescribe, not for the individual; but indiscriminately for the masses, irrespective of individualpreferences. It is a way of coercing patients to take drugs to which many of them strongly object. If artificial fluoridation is so effective then why have scientifically advanced and health conscious countries such as Sweden, Denmark, Norway, Germany, France and Japan totally rejected using it? What is more important is the fact that there is no evidence that children's teeth in those countries are any worse than those in Australia, Canada, Ireland, New Zealand and the United States.

Sadly most dentists are of the mind-set that if fluoridation reduces tooth decay in children, then it is worthwhile. From the legal point of view this is wrong, it is compulsory medication. It is done without the permission of the person on the receiving end.

> *"The incidence of mottled teeth in many developed countries is increasing; at least four well conducted studies have suggested a link between fluoridated water and an increased incidence in hip fractures amongst the elderly"*
>
> Geoffrey E Smith, LDS, RCS(Eng) Dental Surgeon. Dental Research.

Water

> *"The great bulk of evidence from numerous studies therefore supports a link between aluminium consumption, especially monomeric aluminium from drinking water, and an elevated incidence of Alzheimer's disease.*
>
> Harold D. Foster, PHd.2005".

This is a subject that needs to follow on from fluoridation and some comments need to be made about chlorination. I am not trying to scare the pants off you, I just wish to make it clear that there are hazards. There is a minefield out there and you must learn to cross it safely. Hopefully, with me "holding your hand", we can cross it safely together and lead a healthier life. Chlorine certainly kills germs - but what else does it kill? When water is drawn from lakes and rivers rather than underground surface, it comes into contact with soil, silt, mud and effluent. This interaction produces compounds called trihalomethanes (THMs) the most well known being chloroform. Chloroform is a known carcinogen, causing gastrointestinal and urinary tract cancers. Chlorine itself has been linked to high blood pressure, anaemia, arthritis and diabetes and is a contributor to heart disease. Even in a minute quantity sufficient to kill germs, chlorine can undermine the body's defences against artheroscierosis — the hardening and thickening of the arteries.WDDTY,Vo13.No12.

If a plant in your garden fails to grow properly, you may add nutrients to the soil and you will certainly add water. If the water is contaminated you know the plant will be affected. What makes you think this has no bearing on your own health? Clean water is essential to our health. Let's face it we are 80% water. It affects our cells, our enzymatic processes and our ability to detoxify.

Is it possible to name one particular ingredient that is harmful? I don't think so, but it is not difficult to imagine that a cocktail of chemicals could be lethal. The Swedes still blame us for the industrial revolution that precipitated the clouds of acid rain which destroyed fish stocks in their lakes. Falling rain deposits, smoke, dust, chemical fumes, germs, lead and strontium 90 fell on the land. . Rain water then flowed through the soil, flowed into rivers and streams picking up fertilisers and pesticides, as well as herbicides, nitrates and nitrites. We are once again committed to thinking about our cars, and whether we would chose to put the wrong fuel in and expect to get a good performance. Water is so basic to our health that we need to give it very serious consideration.

The simplest and best method to remove contamination is to use a reverse osmosis filter. Having investigated and used various methods of water purification it is reverse osmosis that proved the most satisfactory for me. The backup service is also second to none and the company I use is On Tap Water Supplies, based in Somerton, Somerset. Telephone no 01458274289.

It is not the cheapest method by any means, but to my knowledge it is certainly the most effective as can be seen from the following: The most common impurities measured in parts per million (PPM). I would advise using a multi-mineral supplement to offset any lack of minerals in RO water.

Tap water 400-700 ppm
Jug filtered tap water 275 ppm
Plastic bottled mineral water 175 ppm
Reverse osmosis 6 ppm

So, as you can see a vast difference and I would suggest economical common sense.

In his book *Your Body's Many Cries For Water,* Dr Batmanghelidj recommends that you drink at least two litres of water a day. He also states that dehydration can be responsible for a huge range of ailments and degenerative disease. In the UK now we use sodium fluoride not calcium fluoride for adding fluorine to water. Sodium fluoride is banned in the countries previously mentioned. It was used originally as a rat poison and is a by-product of the aluminium industry.

A detailed review paper published in March 2002 discussed powerful evidence that aluminium from drinking water and other sources was a major contributory factor to Alzheimer's disease.

It was thought for many years that it was impossible for substances to cross the blood/brain barrier. Research now shows that aluminium can react with fluoride in water, and this causes more aluminium to cross the blood brain barrier and deposit in the brain. If there are old pipes in the house then these ought to be renewed, as chemicals deposited from streams can lead to lead, copper and mercury contamination.

So, what is the answer to combat these problems? Bottled and spring water is not the complete answer, as storage in plastic containers for any length of time leads to contamination by synthetic estrogens.

Carbon jug filters are good for reducing chlorine content but not good at leaching out many other contaminants. They also need changing quite frequently.

Ceramic filters are quite expensive but they do remove heavy metals, nitrates, fluoride and bacteria. The weakness is that there is poor removal of organic compounds like pesticides, dioxins and estrogens.

Distilled water. Distillation plants are expensive but they do produce the purest water. It has been suggested that it leaches minerals from the body and the bone structure. I do not think this can be true as thousands of kidney patients using distilled water in dialysis machines show no loss of mineral content in their bodies. Reverse Osmosis. What are the advantages? It is plumbed in with state of the art carbon technology. It uses a membrane under pressure to separate relatively pure water or other solvents from a less pure solution.

Chapter 5

Asthmatic Conditions

This is the most difficult of conditions – distressing, life threatening, and in many cases life shortening. Can it be relieved? Can it be ameliorated? Can it be eliminated? The answer has to be to all those questions – yes! But there are strict guidelines to follow. With my vast experience of this condition, it is only if the patient is committed 100% - total dedication and application that it can be achieved. I have been married to an asthmatic for 25 years – and with all the care and attention she has devoted to controlling this condition, there have been two occasions where emergency shots of adrenaline (Epipen) were administered. That is not a lot over that period of time, but it does point out to you how careful you have to be.

The difficulty is always – which symptoms are apparent on presentation? Is the condition severe? How many times a day is the patient taking drugs? What are they? Are they on steroids? If so, for how long? It goes without saying that if the patient has been on long term cortisone or steroids, it makes the recovery more complicated. However, it can be done, and in many hundreds of cases, it has been. When you are making answers to the questionnaire make sure you list all the symptoms.

On the 22nd March, 2002 a one day conference was held at the Department of Respiratory Medicine in Birmingham Heartland Hospital in conjunction with the Allergy Research Foundation. They discussed the role of nutritional factors, food intolerance and allergy in patients with asthma and put them into the context of management of such patients. Report by Kirsti Peltola, FK, MSc, Nutritional Scientist for the Action Against Allergy magazine.

"Professor Jonathan Brostoff (London) opened the day by reminding the audience about the increasing trends in asthma and deaths from asthma over the last 40 years regardless of the better understanding of the disease mechanisms and treatments. He concluded that there must be other factors, yet not clearly defined, involved in the development of asthma."

"The immediate, true food allergy (IgE mediated) is easy to diagnose, in contrast to food intolerance where the symptoms can be multiple and the time relationship between exposure and effect variable." Professor Brostoff described the role of intact gut mucosa in the development of food allergy and intolerance. If the mucosal membrane of the gut is damaged, there will be an increased permeability through the gut wall allowing undigested food antigens to be absorbed. These antigens can cause the formation of antibodies which will have adverse effects on the body's organs.

Food Intolerance

An indication of the role of food intolerance in asthmatic patients comes from experiments where sodium cromoglycate (it blocks mast cell granulation in the gut and inhibits antigen antigens can cause the formation of antibodies which will have adverse effects on the body absorption) was used to inhibit the food induced asthma attack. Professor Brostoff stressed that *"as very little is known about the role of food allergy and intolerance in other allergic diseases, allergic patients should be treated according to their clinical symptoms rather than adhering meticulously to the mechanism of the disease."*

Professor Brostoff and I go back thirty five years in our association, and I feel sure he will remember the case clearly of Caroline. I am sure, like the Professor, much has been learnt over those thirty five years. Yet, I doubt very much whether either of us has the complete answer. I have to say that in the initial years my major concern was on clearing the lungs and allowing the alveoli to decongest; after all, this was where the major problem lay, or that is what I thought. So, by testing for food intolerance it became clear that dairy products were the major problem and were to be eliminated in total. There is no doubt that many of the asthmatic patients made complete recovery by doing this. However, there were a good many who did not, and even on testing for 'unmasking' (where underlying intolerance had been suppressed by the predominance of the dairy and then came to light) the condition did not improve satisfactorily.

So, even though I was sure I had found the causatory 'trigger', and covered the possible intolerance to various foods, something was eluding me. Professor Brostoff had it in a nutshell when he said, *"if the mucous membrane of the gut was damaged"*. The clue came for me when several asthmatics who had been tolerant of goat and sheep milk originally suddenly found they could not tolerate it any more. Why? The answer had to be a lactose intolerance. Lactose is a sugar. If a patient has a pre-determined candidiasis then the gut mucosa will be compromised and permeability will occur. I can imagine what you are saying – what is a pre-determined candidiasis? I will go in to this condition at some length later in the book, so please bear with me.

In the event we treated the candidiasis by diet and supplementation, put the patients on soya or rice milk and within a very short space of time they recovered. Asthma is a life threatening condition and it is only with total dedication and application that a patient can recover fully. I would suggest therefore, so that too much pressure is not placed on the detoxifying organs, mainly the liver and kidneys, remove the known 'trigger' allergens first. This will allow the adrenal glands to recover as they will have deteriorated to the size of hazelnuts. They will slowly recover to the size of healthy walnuts. This varies with each individual of course, but on average detoxification takes about three weeks, at the end of that period, and you are feeling much better, then consider the diet specifically for candidiasis. I must stress here, that you should not attempt this without guidance from a qualified clinical ecologist. Once you have recovered this is a golden rule you must never ignore. It does not matter how healthy you feel, even though you may no longer need medication

EVEN WHEN YOU FEEL WELL – DO NOT GO ANYWHERE WITHOUT AN INHALER!!

Let me quote a case history. John presented with severe asthma of many years standing, he was taking Ventolin, Becotide, and Becloforte . Approximately every three weeks he was taken in to hospital put on a nebulizer and a heavy course of Prednisilone. John is in his 30's and in business. After his first visit and a full case history and the tests were carried out, he appeared to improve slightly, and he was able to reduce his daily dosage a little. On his second visit a further complication was discovered, and the diet became more severe, however, he found benefit from this, and the visits to the hospital were lengthened to every six weeks or so. On his next visit I questioned John very closely. I asked him to be brutally honest with me. Was he conforming to the dietary strictures the initial testing had placed on him to the letter? The answer was that it was difficult, he bought sandwiches at the office, and it was difficult when he was socialising to keep to the diet. I informed John in no uncertain terms, that if he continued along this path he was not only threatening his own health and immune system, but he was wasting his time and all the effort he was putting in to it. More important to me was that he was wasting my precious time, and I was not prepared to carry on like that. He left after assuring me that he was going to keep strictly to the diet and medication and would advise me of his progress on a weekly basis for a few weeks. Three months later John was off all drugs, feeling wonderful, and running three to four miles a day, with no further hospital visits!

What was the purpose of that case history? Having treated so many hundreds of asthmatics I know only too well, that unless you commit yourself 100% to the programme laid out for you, you are threatening your own life, and wasting yours and my time. Even more important really, you would have been better not to have started the regimen in the first place. If you put additional stress on the adrenal glands, and therefore the immune system, the see saw effect will produce a far more compromised system. With that in mind I wish you well, and to get as much fresh air as possible as often as you can and I wish you a healthy recovery. Perhaps the following letter will encourage you and let you realise what a multi-factorial set of symptoms can be addressed.

Stafford.

Dear Mr Davies,

I am sorry I have not written to you before, but we moved house a few weeks ago, and I have only just caught up with myself! If you remember I brought my daughter Rachel to see you in August (the little girl who said "what's that" before every test). She and I have stuck rigidly to the food that you said we could have, in the face of quite a lot of scepticism especially from my husband. The difference in both of us is quite amazing. Rachel has become much calmer and a nicer child altogether – the child I always ***knew*** *was there underneath. It is no longer a thing to be dreaded when I take her out, and I'll happily let her stay with relatives – who have also noticed the change in her.*

Her attention span has lengthened considerably and she is doing much better at school. She has had no further asthma attacks and has been able to take up ballet lessons which she adores. She has had no further stomach aches, diarrhoea or sickness and I can't thank you enough! She knows herself the difference it has made, and inspects all jars, bottles and packets for ingredients in other peoples' houses as well as ours!

Even her father is coming round to the idea that maybe you were right, and has stopped buying food with additives altogether. Our local Tesco is very good, so there have been few problems. The things we could not get locally such as sweets with no additives ,we ordered from Foodwatch. As far as I am concerned, I had trouble for a few weeks with excruciating stomach pains and constant diarrhoea and headaches. Also a terrible flare up of acne. However, I remembered what you had said, set my teeth and carried on! after about three to four weeks it began to get better. I feel quite good now with a lot more energy than I have ever had before, and more to the point I have had no twinges of arthritis whatsoever, in spite of the cold damp weather. By this time of year I am usually almost crippled with the pain.

Again, many, many thanks for all you have done. All my friends have read your book now and I am definitely spreading the message as far and wide as I can.

Yours sincerely. R.M.C.(Mrs)

The severe reactions of withdrawal that this lady had are typical of someone with a multi-factorial condition.

Diet Sheet for the Elimination of Toxins - Asthma

On rising

Half lemon squeezed into glass of water.

Breakfast

Corn flakes, shredded wheat, puffed rice. Fruit juice (organic), alternative milk.

Tea

Darjeeling, Assam, Luaka. Alternative coffee — Barley cup. Caro. Pionier. (Always read labels for ingredients).

Lunch

Salad — organic if possible. Lettuce. Tomato. Cress. Cucumber.

Celery. Vegetarian cheese cooked). Grated carrot. Grated or shredded cabbage. Beetroot. One or two Ryvita or Matzos crackers. Beef .lamb, chicken . Top fish only. **Not** plaice, dab, or flounder.

Tea

Wholewheat bread and honey. Tea or alternatively coffee.

Supper

Half grapefruit or avocado. Steak, lamb, lamb chops, chicken, cod, whiting, haddock (not smoked), pollock, bream, bass etc. Boiled or baked potato (no skin unless organic), peas, beans, lentils, cabbage, calabrese,broccoli, carrots.

No pork, ham, bacon, veal (unless whey free). No oranges, satsumas, clementines (unless organic). No apple skin, juice, cider or cider vinegar.

YES - Aspalls or Peakes organic apple juice.

This is an elimination of toxins diet for 5 days. After that period you can use safe foods. However, if you are tested further and found to have a pre-disposing candidiasis then the dietary regimen will have to be amended accordingly. I stress once again — under expert supervision. **EVEN WHEN YOU FEEL WELL - DO NOT GO ANYWHERE WITHOUT AN INHALER!**

Chapter 6

Eczema and Skin Conditions

There are some conditions like migraine, where it is possible to point to certain foods as being the causatory 'trigger' for the condition. This is because they have repeated themselves hundreds of times over, making life much easier in correlating the symptoms and the effect. With asthma and eczema this is not the case. Certainly dairy products need to be eliminated in total, but from that point on it becomes much more difficult.

After many years it did become apparent that many cases of eczema in all its forms, had this similarity with asthmatics; there was a pre-disposing candidiasis. I do not think there was one case of psoriasis where this did not apply. I would not recommend that you attempt the candida diet without expert advice. I will list the prime suspects in eczema and it would make sense to eliminate the first listed dairy products then one at a time the foods that follow, you will need at least five days between introducing each food and ascertain reactions.

1. Milk. Butter. Cheese. Rennet. Lactic acid. Casein. Whey, Lactose.
2. Egg yolk, Egg white. Test these separately.
3. Tomato.
4. Peppers.
5. Spices.
6. Additives & Colourings.
7. Sugar.
8. Yeast.

One of the most important things for eczema conditions is to drink as much water as you can. If you can reach the recommended two litres a day then fine. There are indications that using flax oil is beneficial, better when cold and added to food. Cooking destroys much of the omega3 and omega6 essential fatty acids. Remember that topical steroid creams do permeate through the derma and into the bloodstream, It has come to my notice with many patients that when they have been on these for some time bruising becomes a big problem. In some cases the skin breaks as well. The only way I have been able to overcome that is to advise taking a Magnesium Ascorbate in capsule or powder form (3grams daily) with Optizinc 2 daily. After ten days you should notice the bruising becomes less. Then you can reduce the dosage to suit your condition.

London W3

Dear Mr Davies,

Thank you for your letter. I am delighted to report that Jamie's rash has now entirely gone – the digestives are Doves Farm wholemeal biscuits and the contents appear alright. I think one of the juices was bothering him which I've now eliminated and all seems well. He is now his own barometer and when something does slip through we now get an obvious and immediate reaction, which is of course so much easier to cope with. Simon and I can't thank you enough. The horror of much of the last two years is behind us now, thanks to you, and I really dread to think what life would have been like for us all had it gone on undetected.

I always knew that that deep down somewhere in Jamie was a normal, healthy and happy boy, but before your diagnosis began , I only ever was afforded an occasional glimpse, normally when he was out of his routine and not getting the normal amounts of the foods that were bothering him(I now see in retrospect of course). As to my husband Simon, he's been sticking rigidly to your diet and three weeks in there's been no sign whatsoever of a depression – not only that he himself feels so much fitter and a great deal less lethargic.

We will, of course, keep you posted before he sees you again. Once again, our gratitude and many, many thanks.

A & S.K.

How pleasurable to be able to kill two birds with one stone. The son with skin problems and hyperkinesis and the husband with manic depression, who's famous father committed suicide with the same condition. The next condition psoriasis is possibly one of the most complicated of conditions, it usually involves several visits and much detective work, but as you will see by the next letter it is worth the effort.

Nailsea. Avon.

Dear Mr Davies,

Just after Christmas of 1986 I brought my wife, Ivy to see you followed by the usual second visit in March. We take pleasure in writing to advise you of the current situation.

Most of her life suffering from psoriasis and then pustular type and a continual patient at the B.R.I under Dr Waring and then Dr Kennedy, with all the treatments and continually on the varied drugs to control this situation.

Since your discovery of her many allergies and taking up your prescribed diet, to which she adheres rigidly, she has been a different person, with people remarking on how well she is now looking. The final good news that she has been off all drugs completely now culminating in Dr Kennedy discharging her as an out-patient a month ago. The first time in over 40 years.

We are aware that you met Dr Kennedy and given a demonstration, and he is aware that Ivy has visited you and taken up your treatment. She is, of course, continuing to take the vitamins regularly. May we both say how thankful we are to have been put in touch with you – a turning point in her life!

Could you find the time to answer the questions please? What are your views on the possible de-sensitising of allergies? We have heard the odd mention of this here and there – is this a viable proposition when there are so many? Would the tests spoken of spark off an attack of her complaint which, in the past having started would continue through the cycle until completion. Thank you.

Yours sincerely. N.O.

You are sure to be waiting for the answers to those questions so here goes. With such a serious condition it is highly likely that a reaction would occur. There is still not enough evidence to prove that desensitisation is effective. I would not advise it as the allergies are multiple and it would be extremely complicated.

Now to bring you bang up to date November 2010. I had an e-mail from a 3rd generation member of "the family" now residing in Dubai. The 4th generation a girl is suffering with eczema all over her body at eight months of age, so an e mail arrives – can I help? Needless to say I said yes and advised the removal of all dairy products and let me know in five days. The report came back – hooray!! She is clear! But not only that the constipation she was plagued with is now back to normal.

Chapter 7

Depression

Of all the conditions this is the one that gets the least sympathy or understanding. It is human nature to feel sorry for someone who has a plaster on a leg or arm, is in a wheelchair or has scarred features, but very few people have any patience with people with a scarred mind. Unless someone has suffered the black despair on waking to another day, tummy rumbling and butterflies galore, legs shaking and so tearful, it is impossible to put oneself in their shoes. This why I am sure we have all heard people say,"I don't know what is wrong with them, they are so miserable, I wish they would pull themselves together". Or even "I hope they soon grow out of it". What do these sayings mean? Does it mean that they should not be so withdrawn and miserable? Does it mean that they are expected to be bright and cheerful, and be 'normal' whatever that is meant to be? I have not met a depressive yet who would not rejoice at the thought of waking up to a day that held some excitement and they felt 'normal' emotions.

The awful truth is that many of you who suffer from this condition need not necessarily do so. You will have realised that by reading the last letter at the end of the chapter on skin conditions. It is my experience that on numerous occasions it is the effect on the central and para-sympathetic nervous system and the blood/brain barrier brought about by a pancreatic malfunction that contributes to the condition. (Brain Allergies).

Taunton.

Re- appointment booked for 1600 Monday 20th June.

Dear Mr Davies,

As you forecast to me when I visited you for the first time on Tuesday 19th April, I do not need the appointment for the 20th June.

A few weeks after dropping all cow's milk products, tea and white flour products from my diet, the chronic depression has gone! As have also, the pangs of anxiety and periods of feeling troubled and disturbed. A new feeling of confidence and contentment is being experienced daily. Also, too, physical improvements such as clearer skin, shinier hair and believe it or not, a clearer voice has been the result of your guidelines. Only the stomach acidity is unfortunately still with me, but I expect that this will too, in time disappear as did the other symptoms.

As useful side improvements, I have also noticed that short temper and irritability have all but vanished. It seems incredible that all these bad effects have been the result of wrong eating. But there you are the proof is in the pudding'. It only remains, Mr Davies, for me to thank you profusely for having diagnosed the cause of that terrible depression — something that two family doctors and four 'nerve doctors' could not cure or diagnose. That mental blight that started six years ago is gone, completely.

Ich wunsche Ihnen, liebe Herr 'Wunder Doctor' viel Kraft und viel Freunde bei Ihnen Arbeit im Dienste von anderen Menschen. Ich bedanke, ich noch mals bei Ihnen, dags sie mir den Termin am 19 April gegebn haben. Einen recht herlichen Gruss an sie und Ihne Frau sendet Ihnen Ihr

L.P

I must ask you to excuse the last paragraph in German, this man knew I practiced in Germany for many years and he was married to a German lady. In brief he was delighted and thanked me very much. This chap had a manic depressive condition but being married to a German lady he knew that naturopathic or homoeopathic treatments could help. He had reached the point where he was afraid to go out and meet people (agoraphobia). He had trained as a cabinet maker in this country and in Germany but his shaking hands would not allow him to work. He had been told that therapy of various kinds could help but basically "you must learn to live with it". This is not the case and if approached correctly there is often a way out of that black despair.

So what have I found to be the major causatory 'triggers'? I have a feeling that the order of foods to be eliminated will not surprise you.

1. All dairy products.
2. Coffee.
3. Tea bags and tea. Use refined teas as in the Migraine diet. Tea bags invariably contain dioxins.
4. Citrus. Limes, lemons.
5. Tomato.
6. Chocolate in toto. Use Carob.

There are supplements that can help the recovery from depression. But the major factor is getting the diet right. Neurotransmitters are natural substances that transmit messages between nerve cells and the brain. Some neurotransmitters play an important part in regulating our moods. They are serotonin and norepinephrine. The new style anti-depressants like Prozac attempt to regulate serotonin, but a healthy pancreas – sending out all the right messages to the brain soon redresses the problem. In the early stages I would recommend a supplementation of Magnesium ascorbate and B-Complex and possibly phosphatidyl serine. Once you are aware of being stable then you can reduce or even leave these supplements out.

Chapter 8

Gynaecological (Women's problems)

What a wonderful term this is. It covers a multitude of problems that can be experienced by the long-suffering woman. Because I dealt with allergy/food sensitivity it was considered by many of my patients that I did not deal with 'women's problems'.

Let me state now that a pancreatic malfunction can produce all the symptoms previously mentioned and all that I am about to mention. A healthy body, produces a healthy mind, and a healthy hormonal body. Remember that lovely word – Homeostasis. A perfect balance of mind, body and spirit.

One particular instance flies to mind, a lady patient came with a catarrhal problem, she was a very well known local singer, and I have watched many of her performances. During our consultation I mentioned the fact that it was probably the costumes she had to wear, but I thought she was putting on weight. "Yes, I have, it has rocketed on over the last eighteen months, but it is a woman's problem so you can't deal with it". I asked her what made her think I could not deal with it. "Well, you are the allergy man". Yes I am, but I have also dealt with women's problems for as long as I can remember. "What is the problem", I asked. "Oh! I have been bleeding for the last eighteen months, I have seen the doctor and the specialist and I am going to have a full hysterectomy". "Is this what you really want" I asked? "Well, no, but what can you do about it?" When is the operation due? "Three weeks time" she said. "In that case you do not give me a lot of breathing space, but I never give up until the last moment so let us give it a go". I tested her and found there were several things wrong with her diet and gave her Agnus Castus to take daily. *Vitex Agnus Castus* is a cactus from the

Mediterranean

She rang me ten days later from her doctor's surgery to tell me "the doctor has just given me an examination, the bleeding has stopped, and I do not need operative surgery". So much for food sensitivities and Vitex Agnus Castus which I have used for more than twenty years for 'ladies problems'.

Historically ,Vitex was used by the ancient Greeks and Romans to promote chastity. Indeed, this is how the plant gained the name the 'chaste tree', as it was used by monks to suppress sexual desire. Other uses by the ancients included the treatment of injuries, inflammation and epilepsy as shown in Table 1. However, it is the uses of Vitex for women's problems which have persisted to modern times. I have used Vitex for stimulating milk flow in lactating women with great success, but I used it mainly for symptoms in women associated with the menstrual cycle. I say mainly, for there have been several cases where it has been instrumental, along with the elimination of toxins, in correcting hormonal imbalance and inducing fertility and pregnancy in what appeared to be infertile women.

Newton Abbot.

Dear Mr Davies,

I felt I must drop you a line to tell you our good news. Having been sticking to my diet now for 11 months, I do feel so much better and, as you said , the 'other event' would probably happen when my body was better. Well, I'm delighted to say I am now pregnant and the baby is due in May.

We're both delighted but I feel I must write to say thank you to you for your guidance and lovely understanding manner I'm not very good with words but I'm really trying to say a big "thank you".

With very, very best wishes for you and your wife. Keep up the good work.

Yours sincerely

PD

TABLE I

c.400B.C.	Hippocrates recommended Vitex for injuries, inflammation and enlargement of the spleen. Pliny reported diverse indications for Vitex: combating flatulence, diarrhoea and as an antidote to bites from spiders and snakes.
c.A.D.50	Discoroides reported its use for inflammation of the womb and for stimulating mother's milk.
A.D. 1200	In the Persian school, Al-Kindi recommended Vitex for epilepsy.
A.D. 1633	Gerard and other renaissance herbalists recommended Vitex for inflammation of the uterus.
A.D. 1930	Madaus* undertook the first modern clinical trials of Vitex.
A.D. 1953	First clinical work on the galactagogue activity of Vitex.

*German company distributing Homoeopathic/Naturopathic remedies.

Typically the types of condition I have used Vitex for have been PMS (Pre-menstrual tension), oligomenorrhoea (sparse or infrequent menstruation), PCOD (polycystic ovary disease) a hormonal disorder characterized by inadequate secretion of luteinizing hormone, menorrhagia (heavy bleeding), and amenhorrhoea (lack of menstruation). The activity of Vitex has been enhanced by the elimination of toxins (finding the cause). I have a feeling that the inscription on my gravestone will be "he tried to find the cause". But as in the case of any condition, particularly hormonal, you cannot bring about total resolution of the problem unless you find the causatory 'trigger'. With infertility problems and miscarriage I used an adage that I am fairly sure was stimulated by something I read by Rudolf Steiner — "if the soil in the garden is too acid or too alkaline and you then plant the wrong seed or plant — nothing will grow". You must prepare the soil first and get it healthy.

HRT and The Pill.

It has been a long time held belief of mine that to control painful periods, or even acne, young women are increasingly being prescribed the contraceptive pill and antidepressant drugs at a cost to their long-term hormonal and mental health. Whenever I had a lady patient who was on the pill or HRT I encouraged them to accept my philosophy, all drugs have side effects, artificial hormones are no different, they are handy, they control situations, but at what cost? Surely, it must be better to find out why HRT or the pill was necessary. Would it not be better to find out what went wrong and to correct that first? Given a chance, this wonderful body of ours, that on occasions for whatever reason goes awry, will recover remarkably quickly given the right guidance.

There really is a lot of literature about HRT and the Pill which I think you should read, and I will be listing these in the back of the book. It really is mind boggling to me that when problems arise people do not try to find out what caused it or, of more importance, find out what the ingredients are of the drug they are being prescribed. What is in it? Where does it come from? HRT is a classic – where does it come from?

People in Glass Houses

We in the West are quick to condemn the practice in the Far East of imprisoning bears in tiny cages for all their lives in order to extract bile from their gall bladders every 10 days for 'medicinal purposes'. But in recent years a great many women in the West take HRT (Hormone Replacement Therapy) not only to ease the menopause but for the rest of their lives. In fact up to 4 million British women take some form of oestrogen supplement. The most common drugs are PREMARIN and PREMPAK-C produced by a giant factory in Manitoba, Canada. The 'factory' is composed of 45,000 pregnant mares, standing in tiny narrow stalls, unable to move backward or forward or even lie down, strapped with uncomfortable equipment to catch their urine, and with curtailed drinking water to make the urine stronger. The deprived foals, 100 at a time, are sent, in huge sealed containers, 1800 miles to Connecticut slaughterhouses — the eventual fate of their mothers. It is estimated that the number of mares killed in the industry, in Western Canada alone, adds up to 500,000.

But there are cruelty—free HRT options available! So, if any of you reading this would like an alternative to what you are prescribed bear in mind there are 9 alternatives. A full list of these can be obtained from the Hillside Animal Sanctuary, Hall Lane, Frettenham, Norwich, NR12 7LT.

I have to say that I was amazed when I found out how HRT is obtained. I am obviously pleased that there are alternatives but, having said that, I sincerely believe that the right way is to find out why things have gone wrong and correct them. Since I retired I have held training courses for qualified practitioners and I will list these in the back of the book. So, if you have a problem, consult one of them first, and it would be sense to consult your doctor about any anxieties you may have.

I will make a note of recommended books at the rear of this book. As we are on this subject a book that is a must, as far as I am concerned, is one by Dr Ellen Grant who took part in the first major British study of the contraceptive pill in 1961 and is the author of several papers on its effects. She is also an adviser to the Dyslexia Institute and to Foresight — the organisation for the Pre-conceptual Care of Women. Her first book *The Bitter Pill* was an eye opener, but this one (1994) is broader in content and if you wish to understand about hormones and what happens, this is the one. *Sexual Chemistry-Understanding our hormones, The Pill and HRT.*

I mentioned Foresight — what an organisation this is. I am delighted to say that Nim Barnes, the founder, is a friend of mine of too many years standing to mention here. She has worked tirelessly, along with others, to bring expert care and advice to women, young and old, on pregnancy, miscarriage, sexual diseases and the vast subject of 'women's problems'. Her organisation has helped so many patients of mine and I would like to say to Nim in print – a BIG THANK YOU! not just for what you have done in the past but, at the age when most of us are thinking of retiring, you are tireless in pursuing the cause you believe in so passionately. The address of Foresight will be in the back of the book. Also the latest most helpful book will be listed, a must for every mother-to-be.

Premarin

In July 2002 in America a report occurred in Good Medicine, the magazine for members of PCRM, the Physicians Committee for Responsible Medicine. The heading of the article was **The Verdict Goes Against Premarin.** "The Women's Health Initiative which was studying the effects of combined oestrogen and progestin used in postmenopausal women, was halted. It ended three years early after researchers observed an increased risk of breast cancer, potentially deadly blood clots, strokes and heart disease in women taking hormones (compared to those in the placebo group who remained symptom free)."

As I pointed out earlier the withdrawal of these hormones must be done cautiously, but, providing the necessary replacements are instigated at this time, I have never had a problem with my women patients remaining hot flush and menopausal symptom free. I treated many hundreds in this way, but I must stress the dietary regimen was altered also.

Chapter 9

Irritable Bowel Syndrome – Diverticulitis

Crohn's disease – Colitis – Spastic colon

I referred earlier to a one day conference, reported by Kirsti Peltola FK,MSc for Action Against Allergy, where Dr John Hunter (Cambridge), a gastroenterologist, spoke on the mechanisms of food intolerance and presented staggering statistics: 50% of patients referred to gastrointestinal clinics are diagnosed to have Irritable Bowel Syndrome (IBS), a digestive disorder with unknown cause. However, most of the IBS patients are able to date the start of their symptoms to a gastrointestinal infection, prolonged or frequent use of antibiotics or a hysterectomy. These all point to the direction of distorted bacterial flora as a cause of the symptoms, especially overgrowth of facultative anaerobes. Some twenty years ago it was suggested by Dr Hunter and his colleagues that food intolerance may be a major factor in the pathogenesis of IBS. They had looked at the role of high and low fibre diets as a way to treat IBS patients. In their study 67% of patients benefited from a low fibre diet." It is interesting that my findings were exactly the same but I would say that the percentage of patients to benefit from a low fibre diet would be higher than 67%. How I wish that other gastroenterologists would take this on board instead of quite frequently recommending a high fibre diet.

You will note that I have put all these conditions under one heading — **Gut Conditions**. The reason for this is that over the years it became very apparent that there was a great similarity between all of them. So, "we treated that damned impostor just the same".

It is a most distressing condition which if not diagnosed and treated properly can cause the patient to lead their life with one dominant thought to the forefront of their mind. "Where is the nearest loo". I have had patients tell me that they could not go anywhere without planning the route and having a loo available at regular intervals.

What are the symptoms?

Intermittent constipation/diarrhoea, stabbing pains in the gut, bloating after food, hunger that cannot be assuaged, in Crohn's disease there is often blood or mucous in the stool. In some cases food passing through totally undigested.

Birdlip
Gloucestershire
Dear Mr Davies,
I am writing rather belatedly, to thank you for your very effective treatment of my husband's illness — the symptoms of which, as you know, were nausea, chronic stomach pains and total loss of energy.

Before coming to see you, the orthodox medical profession eventually diagnosed the illness as " a nervous tummy which he would have to live with". This diagnosis came after ineffective drug treatment, major abdominal surgery (hernia repair), more internal investigation and a recommendation that further major surgery (gall bladder removal) "might clear the problem. I am happy to say that, by following your advice regarding diet and accepting other non-drug treatment recommended by you, my husband no longer has stomach pain, feels well, and his energy levels are generally back to the normal high.

If you had not been recommended to us by acquaintances I believe that by now my husband would be very poorly indeed. At age 43/44 he changed, from a person full of vitality and with high energy levels, to someone who always felt unwell and who had to make a conscious effort to undertake even normal activities.

This experience has left me in no doubt that there is a serious lack of knowledge (perhaps deliberate — too many vested interests?) in the orthodox medical profession. My husband saw two GP's, a consultant surgeon and a consultant physician re the cause of his illnesses. I believe there must be many more people like him who are suffering unnecessarily, and we both take every opportunity to recommend your treatment.

Thank you again, from both of us, for your excellent medical advice and we wish you continuing success in your work.

Yours sincerely

Marian and Tony S.

I can understand the comments made in that letter; like any loving wife she watched her husband suffer and it would appear that there was no resolution to the problem. But, I must stress, because it is so important, your GP is not to blame, he has not been trained in alternative therapies, his course of action, if he cannot resolve the problem, is to recommend a consultant who has not had alternatives put to him either, he has been trained in the allopathic path as well, which, invariably means drugs or operative techniques, and in many cases these are successful.. The only way that the various therapies can evolve within modern medicine is for discussion. Many are consultants and GPs who have read my books or read Brain Allergies, and have been 'awakened'. I do not feel in any way superior to a GP or a consultant because I can often rectify what appear to be insoluble problems. My training was an osteopath/naturopath/homeopath pathway, then nutritional training and dietary education. Totally different to mainstream medicine. So what I am saying is "don't knock the messenger", at least he has in many cases carried out tests that indicate what the problem is, it is then up to you to decide which avenue you take to rectify it. Then if it is an alternative route, and it is 100% successful, it is your duty to at least tell him or her what has happened. At least that way they may learn something too.

Is there a recommended diet for gut conditions? Yes, the migraine exclusion diet. You will find the majority of symptoms will disappear completely, and if in doubt consult a clinical ecologist.

A word of warning!

Bioflavinoids are invariably citrus unless otherwise stated. Always watch labels carefully – manufacturers change ingredients all the time.

This is as good a time as any to bring to your attention some of the potentially harmful ingredients commonly used by the personal care industry:

Alcohol

A colourless, volatile, inflammable liquid produced by the fermentation of yeast and carbohydrates. Alcohol is used frequently as a solvent and is also found in beverages and medicine. As an ingredient in ingestible products, alcohol may cause body tissues to be more vulnerable to carcinogens. Mouthwashes with an alcohol content of 25% or more have been implicated in mouth and tongue cancers. This is obviously implicated in candida albicans, and in most cases there is pre-disposition to this complaint, causing an imbalance in gut flora.

Elastin of High Molecular Weight

A protein similar to collagen that is the main component of elastic fibres. Elastin is also derived from animal sources. Its effect on the skin is similar to collagen.

Fluorocarbons

A colourless, non-flammable gas or liquid that can produce mild upper respiratory tract irritation. Fluorocarbons are commonly used as a propellant in hair sprays.

Formaldehyde

A toxic, colourless gas that is an irritant and a carcinogen. When combined with water, formaldehyde is used as a disinfectant, fixative or preservative. Formaldehyde is found in many cosmetic products and conventional nail care systems.

Petrolatum

A petroleum based grease that is used industrially as a grease component. Petrolatum exhibits many of the same potentially harmful properties as mineral oil.

Propylene Glycol

A cosmetic form of mineral oil found in automatic brake and hydraulic fluid and industrial anti-freeze. In skin and hair products, propylene glycol works as a humescent, which is a substance that retains the moisture content of skin or cosmetic products by preventing the escape of moisture or water. Material Safety Data Sheets (MSD'S) warn users to avoid skin contact with propylene glycol as this strong skin irritant can cause liver abnormalities and kidney damage.

Alpha Hydroxy Acid

An organic acid produced by anaerobic respiration. Skin care products containing AHA exfoliate not only damage skin cells but the skins protective barrier as well. Long-term skin damage may result from its use.

Glycerin

A syrupy liquid that is chemically produced by combining water and fat. Glycerin is used as a solvent and a plasticiser. Unless the humidity of air is over 65%, glycerin draws moisture from the lower layer of the skin and holds it on the surface, which dries the skin from the inside out.

Kaolin

A fine white clay used in making porcelain. Like bentonite, kaolin smothers and weakens the skin.

SodiumLauryl Sulphate(SLS)

An anionic surfacant used in cosmetics and industrial chemicals as a cleansing agent. Used as a thickener and a foaming agent in shampoos, toothpastes, and cleansers, and as a wetting agent in garage floor cleaners, engine degreasers, and auto cleaning products. SLS is used around the world in clinical studies as a skin irritant. High levels of skin penetration may occur at even low concentrations. Studies have shown SLS to have a degenerate effect on the cell membrane due to its protein denaturing properties. It can also maintain residual levels in major organs of the body from skin contact. Carcinogenic nitrates can form in the manufacturing of SLS or by its combination with other nitrogen bearing ingredients within a formulation, creating a nitrosating agent.

Aluminium

A metallic element used extensively in the manufacture of aircraft components, prosthetic devices and as an ingredient in antiperspirants, antacids and antiseptics. Aluminium has been linked to Alzheimer's disease.

Animal Fat (Tallow)

A type of animal tissue made up of oily solids or semisolids that are water insoluble esters of glycerol with fatty acids.

Animal fats and lye are the chief ingredients in a bar of soap; a cleaning and emulsifying product that may act as a breeding ground for bacteria.

Lanolin

A fatty substance extracted from wool which is frequently found in cosmetics and lotions. Lanolin is a common skin sensitiser that can cause allergic reactions, such as skin rashes.

Lye

A highly concentrated watery solution of sodium hydroxide or potassium hydroxide. Lye is combined with animal fats to make bars of soap, which may corrode and dry out the skin.

SodiumLaureth Sulphate(SLES)

SLES is the alcohol form (ethoxylated) of SLS. It has higher foaming qualities and is slightly less irritating, but may cause more drying. May also cause potentially carcinogenic formulation of nitrates, or nitrosating agents, by reacting with other ingredients.

Bentonite

A porous clay that expands to many times its dry volume as it absorbs water. Bentonite, commonly found in many cosmetic foundations, may clog pores and suffocate skin.

Collagen

An insoluble fibrous protein that is too large to penetrate the skin. This collagen, found in most skin care products, is derived from animal skins and ground up chicken feet. This ingredient forms a layer of film that may suffocate the skin.

Mineral oil

A derivative of crude oil (petroleum) that is used industrially as a cutting fluid and lubricating oil. Mineral oil forms an oily film over the skin to lock in any moisture, toxins and wastes, but hinders normal skin respiration by keeping oxygen out.

Talc

A soft grey-green powder used in some personal hygiene and

cosmetic products, inhaling talc may be harmful as this substance is recognised as a potential carcinogen.

Dioxins

A potentially carcinogenic by product that results from the process used to bleach paper at paper mills. Dioxin treated containers sometimes transfer dioxins to the product itself.

Journal of the American College of Toxicology. Volume 2.

This information is not designed to alarm you, but to make you aware that not everything is quite what it seems. Not only in the food industry but in every industry. For instance in tea bags and more importantly where women are concerned it is used to bleach tampons and sanitary towels. Go to your health shop and get the natural varieties.

Chapter 10

Candida Albicans

When I retired from practice I could almost guarantee that I would see at least four to six patients a day with advanced gut condition and they would on average be below thirty years of age. The amount of teenagers and babies with it, sometimes born with it, increased all the time and, it goes without saying, worried me a lot as it was obvious that we were looking at a condition of almost epidemic proportions. The last chapter on gut conditions is a perfect lead in to candida albicans. This is because so many patients with a compromised gut condition and disturbed gut flora inevitably have candida albicans. You will recall in the earlier chapter on Gut Conditions that Dr John Hunter a gastroenterologist made the comment of staggering proportions that "50% of patients referred to gastroenterology clinics are diagnosed to have IBS (Irritable Bowel Syndrome), a digestive condition with unknown cause". I have reservations about that last statement but it does point out how widespread the condition, amongst others, has become .You will recall also how Professor Jonathan Brostoff referred to the gut permeability problem in association with food intolerance. The one thing I would like to make clear is that I always referred to it as a parasitic condition. It simplifies things and avoids breaking them down to name labelling. As far as I am concerned it is a generalised parasitic condition. I really did not think the patient desired or needed to know whether it was a trophozoite or a helminth, he or she had an upset gut and attendant symptoms. So forgive me if I spend a little time on this subject. Perhaps if I give the explanation of candida it will help.

Candida albicans is a yeast spore which lives in the mucous

membrane of the gut in all of us from the age of six months onwards. The gut flora should consist of 17% candida albicans approximately, the balance being made up by lactobacillus acidophillus, lactobacillus bifidus bifidum and lactobacjllus foetidus. Because it is present in all of us candida albicans tends to be overlooked by physicians seeking the cause of certain conditions. Because of a pancreatic enzymatic malfunction the acid/alkaline balance of the gut becomes acid and the candida proliferates, causing all manner of symptoms which I will list in a moment. Another prominent cause of candida/parasitosis is the overuse of antibiotics, and the preponderance of sugar in the average diet.

DO YOU SUFFER FROM?

Mark as a 5 if the answer is yes.

Depression
Vaginal infections
Anxiety
P.M.T.
Irritability
Menstrual Problems
Heartburn
Athletes Foot
Indigestion
Herpes
Bloating
Cravings for sugar
Fatigue
Cravings for bread
Allergies
Cravings for alcohol
Acne
Joint swelling or arthritis
Migraine

Nasal congestion
Cystitis
Sore throats
Thrush
Wheezing

Have you used?

- Frequent antibiotics (commonly treated with antibiotics)
- The Pill
- A diet high in meat and dairy products

If you can answer "yes' to 10 or more in the first section and more than one in the second section there is a definite possibility that you may have an overgrowth or infection of candida albicans (parasitosis).

I suspect that I would not be far off the mark if I said that most people could find some of those symptoms to complain about. It really is a guide and not to be taken as 'gospel'. A further aid to a practitioner would be to complete the following questionnaire. I would suggest that you complete this, add up your score and then make a judgement as to whether you wish to continue treatment. Obviously my advice would be to consult a Clinical Ecologist for expert advice. However, I am giving you the benefit of all my years in practice. If you follow the guidelines prescribed then you should be fine. Having said that I cannot take responsibility for any procedures adopted and your doctor should be advised.

NUMBER	QUESTION POINTS
1. Have you taken tetracyclines (vibramycin etc) or other antibiotics for acne for one month or longer?	35

2. Have you at any other time in your life taken broad spectrum antibiotics for respiratory, urinary or other infections for 3 months or more or in shorter courses 4 or more times in 1 year?	35
3. Have you taken a broad spectrum antibiotic for one single course?	6
4. Have you, at any time in your life, been bothered with persistent prostatitis, vaginitis, thrush or other problems affecting your reproductive organs?	25
5. Have you been pregnant 2 or more times?	5
1 time	3
6. Have you taken birth control pills — more than 2 years?	15
For 6 months to 2 years?	8
7. Have you taken prednisone or other cortisone based drugs?	
For more than 2 weeks?	15
For 2 weeks or less?	6
8. Does exposure to perfumes, insecticides, fabric shop odours and other chemicals provoke moderate to severe symptoms	20
Mild symptoms	6

9. Are your symptoms worse on damp, muggy days or mouldy places?	20
10. Have you had athletes foot, ring worm, 'jock itch', or other chronic fungus infections of the skin or nails?	20
11. Have such infections been...	
Severe or persistent?	20
Mild or moderate?	10
12. Do you crave sugar in dried fruit form?	10
Do you crave breads?	10
Do you crave alcoholic beverages?	10
Does tobacco smoke really bother you?	10
For each of your symptoms enter point score and total	....
TOTAL	....

SECTION B

For each of your symptoms enter appropriate figure in bracket.

Symptoms mild – 3 pts

More frequent & mildly severe – 6 pts

Severe – **9** pts

Fatigue or lethargy	( )
Feeling of being drained	( )
Poor memory	( )
Feeling 'spaced out' or 'unreal	( )
Depression	( )
Numbness, burning, tingling	( )
Muscle aches	( )
Muscle weakness or paralysis	( )
Pain and/or swollen joints	( )
Abdominal pain	( )
Constipation	( )
Diarrhoea	( )
Bloating	( )
Troublesome vaginal discharge	( )
Persistent vaginal burning/itching	( )
Prostatitis	( )
Impotence	( )
Loss of sexual desire	( )
Endometriosis	( )
Cramps/ Menstrual irregularities	( )
Premenstrual tension	( )
Spots in front of the eyes	( )
Erratic vision	( )

TOTAL SCORE SECTION B ....

SECTION C

For each of your symptoms enter appropriate figure in the bracket .

Occasional or mild 1 point
Frequent/Moderately severe 2 pts
Severe/Disabling 3 points.

Drowsiness	( )
Irritability or jitters	( )
Incoordination	( )
Inability to concentrate	( )
Frequent mood swings	( )
Headache	( )
Dizziness/Loss of balance	( )
Pressure above ears — feeling of head swelling or tingling	( )
Itching	( )
Other rashes	( )
Heartburn	( )
Indigestion	( )
Belching/Intestinal gas/Boating	( )
Mucous in stools	( )
Haemorrhoids	( )
Dry mouth	( )
Rash or blisters in mouth. Mouth ulcers	( )
Bad breath (Halitosis)	( )
Joint swelling or arthritis	( )
Nasal congestion/discharge	( )
Post nasal drip	( )
Nasal itching	( )
Sore or dry throat	( )
Cough	( )
Pain or tightness in chest	( )
Wheezing or shortness of breath	( )

Urgency/frequency of urination	( )
Burning on urinating(cystitis)	( )
Failing vision	( )
Burning or tearing of eyes	( )
Sand in eyes feeling	( )
Recurring infections or fluid in ears	( )
Ear pain or deafness	( )

TOTAL SECTION 'A'
TOTAL SECTION 'B'
TOTAL SECTION 'C'

GRAND TOTAL SCORE ....

The Grand Total Score will help you and your physician decide if your health problems are connected. Scores in women will be higher than men as 7 items in the questionnaire apply exclusively to women, while only 2 apply to men.

Yeast connected health problems are almost certainly present in women with a score over 180. Men with a score over 140.

Similar problems are possibly present in women with a score of over 120. Men with a score over 90.

Although lessened there is a possibility of a yeast connection with scores as low as women with a score of 60. Men with a score of 40.

WITH SCORES OF LESS THAN 60 WITH WOMEN AND 40 IN MEN YEAST RELATED PROBLEMS ARE CERTAINLY LESS LIKELY.

The symptoms in Section "C' commonly occur in patients with yeast related problems they are also found in patients with other conditions.

The more I have looked into, and treated, the parasitic problems afflicting a great number of patients, the more I realise that I could write a book on this one subject alone. There have been many books written on this subject and I will name some in the back of this book but I am not yet aware of anyone who has written about the subject objectively with **clinical report back results.**

In 1997 I sent out a questionnaire to 500 of my patients known to have a predisposing candidiasis/parasitosis. The results were quite surprising.

TAKING A BROAD SPECTRUM ANTIBIOTIC - 263
AFFECTED BY TOBACCO SMOKE - 218
SUFFERING VAGINITIS/THRUSH ETC - 185
PREGNANT 2 OR MORE TIMES - 176
DO YOU CRAVE BREADS - 169
AFFECTED BY DAMP MUGGY DAYS - 159
HAVE TAKEN BROAD SPECTRUM ANTIBIOTICS - 153
DO YOU CRAVE SUGAR - 142
BIRTH CONTROL PILL 2 YEARS - 139

The highest % of answers to all groups was in the 30-39 age group.

The second highest was in the 20-29 group.

It is fairly conclusive going by these figures that the over prescribing of antibiotics is one of the primary causes of an imbalance of gut flora.

It is interesting to note on the Database that the questions answered in the highest percentages were:

FATIGUE OR LETHARGY SEVERE 75%
FEELING OF BEING DRAINED SEVERE 83%

It is therefore my hypothesis that those suffering from Myalgic Encephalomyelitis (ME) were suffering from, and this proved to be the case, a pre-disposing parasitosis. When stool samples were provided, in every case either Ebstein Barr Virus or Cytomegalovirus were implicated. No wonder then that their major complaint was the total lethargy and being constantly drained. The overall conclusion for me was that there was a total Gut Dysbiosis(Imbalance).

This is such a serious subject that obviously we must go in to it further. But perhaps it might be a good idea to inject a sense of humour here. One young lady who was extremely poorly but with an obvious sense of humour sent me the following: (Bear in mind please that I am a 'golf nut' and of Welsh origin).

G od Davies, he'll sort out your pain. Welsh name but no accent,ah!whatashame.

W hether brittle nails or pain in a part, Its all in a days work, this man is all heart.

Y outhful or ancient and all ye in between, get thee to him he's clinically green.

N o time for wasters, raise his ire not a jot, for he'll take a verbal swipe at your bot.

N ow your allergic to flour and cream, such culinary delights are now but a dream.

E xquisite fragrance of garlic so rare, nothing to do with parfumiers' flair.

D on't be disturbed if results are slow to be won. He'll recommend gelignite to stick up your bum.

A nxious that you should be free from all pain, he will request that you visit again.

V aliant struggles ensue from now on, beware of the food devil waiting anon.

I f in doubt, telephone, you always could. Dear God! It's Natalie – Victoria Wood!

E xceptional doctor, a talent sublime. Medical mountains with him you will climb.

S o now it's off to improve handicap
Don't break a leg or you'll land in the BUNKER!

You may have gathered that this dear girl, as ill as she was, was called Natalie. She had a sense of humour that reminded me so much of Victoria Wood, I used to tell her of this. The reference to breaking the leg is because I slipped on the 14th hole one morning, a week before my wedding, and broke my leg. Anyway, I hope you enjoyed that little moment of the sublime. Now back to the serious stuff.

The following is an extract from *Women Alive — Awareness Is Life* —1995 by Lisa Mark PA-C. "*Candida Esophagitis. An infection frequently underestimated in HI V infected Women is Candida Oesophagitis, (a yeast infection in the oesophagus). It is closely related to thrush (a yeast infection in the throat) and Candida vaginitis (a yeast infection in the vagina) and the only difference is its location in the oesophagus — the tube that connects the mouth with the stomach. In one study patients at risk for AIDS were found to have Candida oesophagitis as the only initial opportunistic infection.*

Candida albicans is the most common fungus (yeast) in people with AIDS.

The majority of women with oesophageal candidiasis also have oral thrush. There is a national debate going on over whether there is an emerging resistance to antifungals, especially orals, from using medications like Diflucan, too early in the course of HIV It is not clear whether using Diflucan and others for fungal prevention actually improves or increases one's life or if it creates greater problems'.

Because parasitosis has become a major source of enlightenment over the last ten years, it was quite noticeable that practitioners were treating the condition as the answer to everything; treating accordingly. It certainly is far more common now, and we, as practitioners, need to be aware. Having said that my approach would always be as follows. The patient's immune system, judging by the symptomology, will have been severely compromised and the organ that will be attempting to cope with the toxins will be the liver.

Many patients describe their symptoms as feeling "liverish"; indeed some do have a very sallow complexion. What you should not do is rush in and treat the parasitosis immediately. This applies particularly to the younger age group - generally speaking their immune system is more responsive and therefore more reactive.

What Procedure

The first thing to do is to test for food hypersensitivities and eliminate these for three weeks. At the end of that time check which symptoms remain. If it is obvious that there is a parasitosis still manifesting, then commence the treatment plan for three weeks and assess the situation then as to the next step.

Is it worth doing a stool test?

The short, sharp answer to that after years of carrying out these tests, by sending a stool culture away, is, "No". For some years I had the results from these tests and, although I had tested for and diagnosed candidiasis, the results were coming back – negative! Without wishing to sound big headed I considered myself to be a very good diagnostician, so these stool results were not ringing true. So I rang the laboratory and chatted to the headman. I was much relieved when he assured me that I was one of dozens that had the same anxiety.

Misdiagnosis? "No", he said, "You would need to send me a stool culture every day for at least seven days for me to get a true result, the various stages of encystation that takes place when everything is active would be somewhere in that time scale". So, I decided to rely on my own observations, symptomology, and the questionnaire and I have to say this proved to be far more accurate and successful than the stool test, which carried out privately was quite expensive.

Then of course there is the dilemma of which treatment plan is going to be the most effective. This organism is extremely resilient and difficult to rid from the body. However, the yeast form is not nearly so troublesome as the fungal form. So, if possible catch it early and the success rate will be higher. Once it gets to the fungal form various programmes need to be adopted. Just to give you some idea of the difficulties involved there are approximately 900 species of yeast existing similar to that used in bread making.

What are the most common sites?
Vagina — mouth — gastro-intestinal tract — lungs.

The climate of the vagina is the ideal site for yeast proliferation. It will always head for the wettest, warmest places. Athlete's foot is a classic example of a fungal infection in a warm, often wet, site. I have seen many lady patients who are heavily bosomed and the perspiration beneath has encouraged fungal infection. There are very few patients with severe eczema who have not had a pre-disposing candidiasis. Another common site in men is in the testicular area, commonly referred to as 'jock itch'. The other common site is around the anus where itching can be quite severe. Please do not attempt to use creams or lotions to suppress this condition. It must be treated from whence it came – internally!

The human body is full of micro-organisms competing for nourishment. When the body is healthy and properly maintained, a harmonious balance is maintained. After death, yeast organisms instigate the work of decomposition – a task most of us would rather postpone, I think. Out of the many hundreds of patients I treated for candida/parasitosis, I would say that three out of four lady patients had more than one episode of infection.

It will not surprise you when I say that faulty nutrition is the biggest cause. That is not just my opinion; it is in every book I have read, or medical treatise. Only this morning my wife and I were in a large supermarket and observed a young mother, with the youngster sitting on the trolley eating a lollipop. The trolley was loaded to the brim — but did not contain one item of fresh vegetables or fruit! I guarantee that almost every item in that trolley was full of sugar. What activates yeast? — Sugar. In his book The Encyclopedia of Natural Medicine, Michael Murray cites the following statistics. "In one year the average American consumes: -

- 100 lbs of refined sugar.
- 300 cans of soda pop.
- 200 sticks of gum.
- 18 lbs of sweets and candy.
- 63 dozen doughnuts.
- 50 lbs of cakes and biscuits.
- 20 gallons of ice cream."

I would say that the average person in this country in this year of 2010, is the same, or even more indulgent than the above figures. The biggest culprits are not you, the purchaser, manufacturers have no compunction in using salt and sugar totally unnecessarily.

The human body/pancreas was not designed to cope with those amounts of sugar. Yeast metabolises sugar and produces ethanol — acetaldehyde — and carbon dioxide as chemical by-products. Certainly one of the facts that became patently obvious with this condition was that every patient tested had a vitamin/mineral deficiency.

What are the nutrient destroyers? See also Chapter 14

- Aspirin destroys - Vit **A-** calcium — potassium — **B** Complex — Vit C.
- Caffeine destroys - B1- inositol — biotin — potassium —

zinc.

- Chlorine destroys Vit E.
- Chocolate contains caffeine and fat.
- Fluoride destroys - Vit C.
- Sedatives destroy folic acid - Vit D.
- Menstruation -iron -B12 - calcium -magnesium.
- Stress destroys all vitamin/mineral stores.
- White sugar and flour - B complex.

Antibiotics prescribed and also added to animal feed destroy vitamin stores and create an imbalance. This in turn creates a continual battle for the immune system to remain stable.

When you take antibiotics you not only kill the bad bacteria but the good as well. It is rare that you will hear a physician discussing the fact that one side of antibiotic therapy is the disruption of good intestinal bacteria. Be assured that when healthy bacteria are destroyed there is **always** a price to pay! How many times have I heard lady patients telling me that when they took a course of antibiotics they suffered with thrush.

Which foods to eliminate

I must stress this is the plan I used and **should not be undertaken** without supervision.

All sugars (dextrose, sucrose, maltose, lactose. fructose and maltodextrin) and yeast.

All fruit except for **apple, pear and banana**. You must be tested to make sure these are safe.

Melon, marrow, courgette, swede, parsnip and cooked carrot.

Safe foods for Candida/ Parasite Cleanse

WHENEVER POSSIBLE USE ORGANIC AND FRESH FOODS. YOU ARE TRYING TO STIMULATE HEALTHY CELL STRUCTURE.

YES FOODS

All green fresh vegetables, sweet corn (preferably baby corn as there is less mould).

Basmati white rice.

White flour.

Quinoa, cous cous and semolina.

Sea salt.

FIRST pressed, **COLD** pressed extra virgin olive oil.

Flax oil (Linseed) Hemp oil (Add these to steamed food after cooking).

Drink only bottled water. Reverse osmosis water is fine but make sure the filters are in date.

2 pieces of fruit daily, peeled, **NOT COOKED.**

Organic tea bags are allowed such as Organic Clipper but it is better to use a good quality leaf tea such as Assam, Darjeeling or Luaka (An infuser saves mess). NOT FRUIT TEAS.

Provamil (unsweetened organic soya milk). All soya products should be organic as they could be GM (genetically modified).

NO SOY SAUCE OR VINEGAR.

Lentils and pulses must be soaked in Vit C powder *(magnesium ascorbate)* before cooking to kill moulds. Alfalfa, mung and aduki beans sprouted at home. Remember to wash them through thoroughly morning and night each day.

Soda bread is ideal but watch out for commercial soda bread as invariably they have yeast or milk in them. Use llb organic white SR flour, or spelt flour (which is more nutritious) half pint of water, pinch of sea salt and 1 tablespoon of flax oil. Mix quickly and place in hot oven until cooked through (approx 20 minutes). Longer in a loaf tin.

NO TO THESE FOODS

Do not use mange tout, peas, cucumber, marrow, courgette or any of the squash family.

Initially do not use whole wheat flour as the endosperm

retains moulds and residual pesticides and sprays.

Homeopathic remedies are invariably dextrose or lactose based. Tinctures are alcohol based. Order aqueous tinctures. (Use within 5 days).

Products including cider vinegar. All fruit juices are fermented. Home juicing and drunk immediately are allowable using apple, pear and banana.

Initially watch tomato as it comes under fruit family and is acidic.

No cooked carrot as they convert to high content of sugar.

On the subject of homoeopathic remedies, whilst typing the above, I was reminded just how careful one has to be. A gentleman came to see me who worked in London and Amsterdam; he presented with quite a multi-factorial symptomology and was taking two homoeopathic remedies. These were recommended by one of the top homeopaths in the world. To protect her identity we shall call her Helga.

I did not wish to interfere with her treatment, it was compatible with what we were doing, and he was returning to see her a fortnight later, I asked him to mention that he was on a candida diet and to check that the remedies were not dextrose or lactose based. He returned to see me six weeks later.

I asked him about the remedies and asked "was Helga quite happy about the bases?" Her reply staggered me, "Oh! Don't worry about that. There is such a small amount it is not worth considering". Whilst he was with me, and with his permission, I rang Helga, reiterating what he had told me. She then repeated what she had told him. I said, "Helga, you are recognised as one of the top homeopaths in the world and yet in one short sentence you have just told me and your patient, that homeopathy does not work! Surely you do not mean that? She had completely missed the point and was most apologetic and assured me she would never make that mistake again.

If someone of that eminence can make a simple mistake like that then you will understand why I harp on all the time about you being careful. We all make mistakes. I just wish to ensure that you do not make them, as they can be costly and painful.

Leaky gut

When candida/parasitosis is allowed to proliferate, it can perform an astonishing metamorphosis, changing from a simple yeast cell into a much more harmful "mycoelial" fungal form. Under the microscope, the cell appears to sprout roots and branches; these burrow their way into the walls of the intestine and ultimately can spread throughout the whole body with potentially widespread adverse effects. The most insidious damage is to the gut lining with an increase of toxins called polyamines, which attack the mucosal cells of the gut wall. The outcome of that is "gut permeability", commonly referred to as leaky gut. This allows toxins and undigested food molecules to pass through.

Supplementation

I would like to make it clear that there are many good firms providing supplements but I found after many years that the products that suited me best, and were very effective were those supplied by Biocare Ltd. There are many cheaper products of the same name available, but value for money without being packed with padders and fillers Biocare is the firm of choice. Tel 0121 4333727. Once the initial detoxification diet has been carried out and you are starting the candida diet in earnest then take Oregano complex - 2 capsules daily with food or as directed. This contains freeze-dried grape seed oil, freeze-dried borage oil, freeze-dried oregano oil, freeze- dried wormwood oil *(artemesia absinthium),* freeze-dried ginger grass oil and Vitamin E.

I included the ingredients here to highlight the wormwood. If you enquire at a specialist nursery you should be able to purchase *artemesja absinthjum* plants. They are not expensive. They have attractive grey leaves and grow to approximately three feet high with a two-foot spread. The reason I mention this is that when picked fresh from the plant the leaves are far more effective than any capsule. The leaves can be chewed or in my case, being a coward, placed in a capsule.

This will start the process of destroying the fungal form and after ten days I would introduce Lactobacillus acidophilus from Biocare to replenish the gut flora. It will contain one billion viable cells per dose. **It must be refrigerated once opened** and should have an expiry date. It will be accompanied by a full technical support and information service. Ask for the powder not the capsules. Take as directed by practitioner. I have found that with little babies, patients with severe myalgic encephalomyelitis and those who have a history of problems since early age it is advisable to start with *Lactobacillus bifido bifidum* for a few weeks, as this has been destroyed in the gut, then for a week Lactobacillus bulgaricus and then for approx three weeks the *Lactobacillus acidophilus*. In some of these patients it is necessary to complete a course of a product called Replete, again from Biocare. This is an Intensive Intestinal Re-colonisation Therapy and there is an accompanying BioMed Newsletter No.10 that will give you all the information you need. There have been reports of patients having a headache and quite nauseous for a day or two; this quickly passes so do not worry about it.

Is that it?

Sadly, as I said earlier, this is a complicated condition. We are all as different as our fingerprints or DNA. If there are still symptoms after the previous procedure has been carried out, it may be necessary to proceed with the herbal parasite programme (HPP). Because it has worked so well for my patients, my family and myself, I will not bore you with all the details here. I suggest you buy or get from the library, *The Cure for All Diseases* by Dr Hulda Regehr Clark, Ph.D., N.D. ISBN 1-890035-01-7. Page 338. This will give you all the information you require.

The major thing to remember is that it is a complicated condition, it will take patience and strict adherence to diet — **If you cheat — you cheat yourself.**

Chapter 11

Myalgic Encephalomyelitis

When the last reprint of *Overcoming Food Allergies* was printed in 1998 I used the following as the opening of the chapter. "This has become a very 'popular' condition. Anyone who has a penchant for feeling ill seems to climb on the band wagon, claiming a legitimate excuse for feeling ill, or wanting to feel ill. Hypochondriacs unite. A recent television programme on the subject was presented by an eminent and likable lady doctor. In the past I have always had the greatest respect for this lady. Her programmes were well researched and fairly presented. In this instance, sadly, this does not appear to be the case at all and she ridiculed the disease as being psychosomatic. The programme was subsequently covered by Right to Reply and Clare Francis and others replied in full."

It is now 2010 and little has changed except that it is now recognised as a genuine medical condition, invariably referred to as CFS - Chronic Fatigue Syndrome or PVFS – Post viral fatigue syndrome.

It is interesting to read a BBC report dated 02/05/2010.

"The cause of ME cannot be explained by other conditions, such as depression, and it does not improve substantially after periods of rest. It is estimated that 250,000 in the UK have the condition. Anyone can get it, although it is thought to be more common in women, who make up as much as 75% of cases. The condition usually develops in the early twenties to mid-forties. Children can also be affected, most commonly between the ages of 13-15. The condition has been controversial and it took a long time for the condition to be recognised fully by doctors, and in some circles was

dismissed as 'yuppie flu'. While some remain unconvinced of its existence , it is fully established in the mainstream as a bona fide medical condition."

In every ME case that I treated it was obvious that their immune system had broken down; they were in Stage 3, the adrenal glands were exhausted and they were vitamin and mineral deficient. But significantly, as with many other labelled conditions, it soon became apparent that there was a pre-disposing candidiasis/parasitosis. Once the initial food sensitivities/ allergens were eliminated the symptoms became much clearer and, once treatment commenced, it was amazing how quickly they recovered. It goes without saying, I hope, that strict dietary guidelines are necessary and recovery is slow but the main thing is that recovery is attainable. Keep to the guidelines laid out for candida and the supplementation mentioned. As soon as the symptoms are coming under control, then make sure you take a recommended vitamin/ mineral supplement.

All the conditions I mentioned in the preamble are labels, enabling the medical profession to pigeonhole the condition, and in many ways painting a picture mentally of what is happening. I will be remembered, I am sure, for 'harping' on about the causatory 'trigger'. You can hang on as many labels as you like but until you go back to basics and ask the most important question of all, "Why? How did this illness come about?", then the patient will be the one who loses out as well as the practitioner. He or she will not have the satisfaction I had of seeing patients, who could hardly walk and some who had to be helped up my stairs, coming back some months later bounding up the stairs like spring chickens. The feelings of satisfaction and achievement are tremendous.

Myalgic Encephalomyelitis is another complicated condition and I am not suggesting that you try and do this on your own. Your GP should be informed and you should be consulting a

Clinical Ecologist. Needless to say if you consult one that has been trained by me, you know the procedures will be the same. YOU DO NOT HAVE TO LIVE WITH IT!

Chapter 12

Superbugs

Because of all the notice that is being brought to public attention, almost weekly, in the tabloid press you might think that this is a modern phenomenon. As long ago as 1995 Geoffrey Cannon published a large tome called Super-bug — Natures Revenge. I will list this with other books at the back of this book. For those of you who care about your own health and, as a practitioner, the health of others, this is a book you must read. I would like to just quote from the flyleaf of this book, *"We may look back at the antibiotic era as just a passing phase in the history of medicine, an era when a great natural resource was squandered and the bugs proved smarter than the scientists"*. Professor Ken Harvey (Medical micro-biologist).

Sadly this is now the case. How often on the news now do we hear that a ward in a hospital has been closed due to a 'superbug' or 'super virus'? In our local paper *The Somerset Gazette* on Friday, December 20th 2002, the headline was "Super-bug Shock at Musgrove". It continued, "One patient a day contracts the MRSA super-bug at Taunton's Musgrove Hospital, it was revealed this week. Questions are being raised about hygiene at the hospital after it was disclosed that ten people died there from the antibiotic-resistant disease this year alone."

In the *Daily Mail* on June 13th 2000 Jenny Hope, Medical Correspondent, reported, "Hospital infections are wreaking havoc in wards around the world. Now another deadlier strain has been discovered. The World Health Organisation said that only a handful of cases of the infection, known as VISA, had so far been reported from Britain and world wide but the WHO's Dr Rosamund Williams said that the infection had the potential to explode. In Britain alone there are at least 100,000 cases of hospital-acquired infections each year. As well as the 5,000 who die, the infections are a contributory factor in deaths of 15,000 other patients, with infected patients seven times more likely to die than those who are not struck down." The article continues but enough said.

MRSA – Methicillin Resistant Staphylococcus Aureus

Daily Mail Friday 4th October 2002. Beezy Marsh, Medical Reporter, wrote, *"The Super-bug Surge. Hospital infections are heading for an all time high. The number of deadly 'super-bugs' lurking in NHS hospitals will hit an all time high this year amid growing concern about filthy wards and sloppy hygiene procedures. Britain already holds the shameful title as the "MRSA capital of Europe".*

It was reported in the *Daily Mail* on Saturday 7th December 2002 that the drug to combat these super-bug infections had failed. Linezolid also known as Zyvox had proved ineffective.

I am sorry to say that those type of headlines continued throughout 2002 and now again in 2010. Remember the first report by Jenny Hope was in June 2000. So at least 10 years have gone by and it would appear that the drugs such as Vancomycin, which were kept in reserve to deal with these super-bugs, has also become non-effective. The super-bugs have won the day, as forecast in Geoffrey Cannon's book.

Quite frightening really as it is inclined to put one off going in to hospital. Will it encourage you to take care of your own health? It is a **Wake Up Call**! It is quite normal to hear the comment, "Oh! If we listened to everything you hear and believed everything we read, we would not be able to eat anything." When you read headlines that have been appearing in the press in recent times, that attitude is not surprising: *Daily Mail,* Monday 5th February 2001, Sean Poulter reported, ***"FOOD POISONING HITS OVER 8 MILLION A YEAR.*** *Shock study shows epidemic may be nearly twice as bad as official figures. The* *campylobacter bug is now the biggest single source of poisoning in the UK. Surveys by the Food Standards Agency have found that more than nine in ten fresh and frozen chicken are contaminated with campylobacter and 94.5% of the 13 million pigs slaughtered in the UK in the past year tested positive for the bug. Campylobacter is associated with the normal signs of food poisoning, including upset stomach and loss of fluids, which can be extremely serious for the elderly, sick, young or mothers-to-be. In a few cases it can cause life threatening secondary illnesses such as Guillain-Barre syndrome which brings on total temporary paralysis".*

At least fifteen years ago I was warning patients to be very careful when cooking chicken. In those days salmonella was the worry. Some of you may have seen the TV programme where they illustrated a couple having chicken for lunch. The lady washed the chicken and put it on the draining board while she got the cooking tin. Her husband then wiped the surface with the dishcloth; this spread the campylobacter until most of the kitchen was rife with it on testing. You really must be extremely careful and make sure you cook it through thoroughly.

So is beef a problem because of BSE? Lamb a problem because of scrapie? Pigs a problem because of campylobacter? And chicken - well, it would appear that is totally out of the question.

So what do you eat? One thing is for sure, I am glad I became a vegetarian approximately 12 years ago. That does not solve the problem though because people like eating meat as a general rule. All in all, eating becomes quite a problem in itself. The best you can do is try and find organic meat and truly free range chicken or organic.

It is my opinion that nothing will change very much until the animal husbandry is altered. Mass production has become the order of the day, and we, as the consumer, are the ones who are worst affected. The government have done a u-turn on changing the laws on battery chicken production. The mass producers have yet again won the day; we, the public, will continue to line their purses while the animals suffer horrendous conditions. I wonder if one day the government appointed Food Standards Agency will set a standard and abide by it and not give in to commercial pressure?

What can we do?

The first priority is to shop carefully, secondly cook thoroughly and thirdly do not keep cooked food and raw food together.

One of the most serious gut problems is cryptosporidium and in a lot of medical literature is referred to as 'extremely difficult to cure'. During my practice life I had several patients with this condition and they had been told to 'live with it'. It is recognised as an important cause of infection in both immune-compromised and in otherwise healthy subjects. It can be a pathogen of life threatening potential for AIDS patients. There had to be a way of treating these patients and those affected by MRSA and other super-bugs.

I came across an article on the revival of a centuries old remedy called colloidal silver. Soon after an article by Simon Cave appeared in a national newspaper, "Could a silver drink beat all antibiotics? A solution containing one of our most highly prized metals, silver, is being heralded as the latest alternative to antibiotics. Research has shown that silver suspended in water kills virtually all bacteria, viruses or fungi — even if they are exposed to only minute traces of it. The solution, known as colloidal silver, has been shown in laboratory experiments to kill more than 650 *disease* organisms, whereas most antibiotics kill only about six.

Vitally, it could have an impact on the battle against antibiotic resistant super-bugs such as MRSA and methycillin resistant staphylococcus aureus. Infected patients can become severely ill and even die because the antibiotics don't work against it. Colloidal silver, an odourless yellow liquid with a faint metallic taste, was favoured by the Greeks and Romans. Earlier this century it was used by doctors to treat septicaemia, whooping cough, cystitis and shingles. But when antibiotics were discovered, clinical uses for silver were discarded and it is only recently that its benefits are being rediscovered. Available from most health shops, it can also be applied externally to skin conditions such as acne, eczema and ringworm as well as to burns, cuts and grazes. However, a report in the Journal of Toxicology and Clinical Toxicology warns against the indiscriminate use of silver products and says that there is a lack of information about its effectiveness and potential toxicity."

I first used colloidal silver, along with the elimination diet, and Lactobacillus-acidophillus on the aforementioned patients with cryptosporidium. They began to feel better within days and subsequent visits to the hospital for fecal testing showed no sign of the disease.

A GP colleague of mine from Yeovil rang to say that his mother-in-1aw had contracted MRSA and was being sent home for them to care for; but don't hug her or kiss her and keep the children away from her. As she had a severe rodent ulcer on her right leg there was a possibility that amputation may be necessary. Could I help? To cut a long story short, she recovered splendidly; the ulcer disappeared with homoeopathic cream and colloidal silver dressings within weeks. She went back to her home up North and lived for a good few years after that. She was in her eighties.

My mother-in-law was in a local nursing home and one of her problems was a severely clawed hand (arthritis); the nails punctured the skin and gangrene set in. The home rang to say that the doctor had called and suggested hospitalisation and amputation. As you can imagine, my reaction was, "Not until I have had a go *first.*" I went straight up with a bottle of colloidal silver and asked the staff to give her a teaspoon morning and night and to bathe the hand with the silver three times a day.

Within 24 hours the smell of decay had gone and within three days the hand was back to a normal condition. Subsequently the hand was bathed once a week and the problem has not recurred.

For which conditions can it be used?

Any condition that would normally need antibiotics taken with Lactobacillus-acidophillus to replenish healthy gut flora if taken internally. **When opened please ensure that you keep the probiotic refrigerated. I** would advise you to see a practitioner if the condition is chronic and you would no doubt be recommended to take a liver support as well. I can honestly say that with the many patients I have prescribed this colloidal silver not one adverse comment has been made - only wonderment at how effective it is - and, what is more, it is not expensive. I would recommend everyone to keep a bottle in the medicine cupboard. It even helps with the common cold. *Vis medicatrix Naturae* — the healing power of nature. (Hippocrates) .

Having said all that it may sound as if I am backtracking slightly, actually the opposite, I am advancing ad keeping up to date. It is now possible to obtain Ionic Silver which has taken my wife and I through quite a severe winter without a cold, most unusual! This is available from Wellbeing.research@virgin.net, I will put full contact details in the useful addresses appendix.

Chapter 13

Cancer — The Modern Scourge

In a book by Phillip Day, *Why We're Still Dying to Know the Truth,* he reports the work of Professor John Beard, an Edinburgh embryologist, who, at the turn of the 20th century, demonstrated that cancer was a healing process that had not terminated and that this was **primarily** due to a deficiency of digestive (pancreatic) enzymes, which are used by the body to chew off the protein coating of healing (trophoblast) cells to allow their destruction by the immune system. In the event that trophoblast is not destroyed upon completion of the healing task, the ongoing proliferation of these healing cells will produce tumour mass at the site of the original damage. Beard, of course, had identified the primary role of toxins and carcinogens as being responsible for damaging the body in the first place, triggering a stem-cell reaction.

Forgive me for highlighting those items but it does bear out my hypothesis - or was it mine? - I certainly had not read this book before and I was not aware of Beard's work. But it does point out to you what I said at the very beginning of this book, "The pancreas is the instigatory endocrine/exocrine organ of the body." Ignore it and its malfunction at your peril.

I have treated just about every type of cancer there is but I do not treat the various types a different way; I do not treat any condition differently. I find the instigatory causatory 'triggers' eliminate them, make sure there are no outstanding symptoms and treat them. The body, no matter the condition, will heal itself with a little help from supplementation.

On testing many cancer patients over a period of time it became very clear that in every case there was a predisposing candidiasis/parasitosis. Then I remembered reading in a book many years previously, I think it was by Dr Nadia Coates at the Springhill Cancer Centre, that all cancer cells contained bacteria and fungi – kill the fungi and the body's immune system will kill the bacteria. This appeared to work every time and many patients, who were given a very short time to live, some, many years later are still going strong.

Olney
Bucks
Dear Mr Davies,
I have been meaning to write for some time concerning my father Mr Matthews who came to see you in April 1989 diagnosed with terminal cancer of the spine and pelvis.

You told him cancer was not "fire proof' and suggested the exclusion diet, EDTA and Germanium. He had hardly been able to walk when he came to see you. After the consultation Dad decided, as you know, to forego traditional treatment and stick with it. Within a week of being on the diet he was walking to the town centre a mile from my house.

He lived a happy healthy life as you are aware for twenty-one months and eventually died of bronchopneumonia on 30th November 1990, a week after falling from a step ladder at home.

Of course this was a terrible blow, after all the work that had gone into Dad keeping himself going. I think my sister-in-law phoned to tell you Dad had died. The reason I am writing, however, is to let you have a copy of the post-mortem certificate, which does not indicate any sign of cancer in the vital organs. This gives us hope that the mental and physical efforts Dad made to keep going were in fact keeping the cancer at bay. As mainstream doctors could only offer relief of pain, twenty-one months of virtually pain free living seems like a bonus and who knows how long he might have survived if the accident had not happened.

I know you are keen to keep in touch with the progress of

patients and, although this is, as ever, anecdotal evidence, it does prove that where there was no hope — hope was found.

I would have written to you earlier; I'm afraid it has taken this long as there has been quite a lot going on since Dad died.

I hope you find this information useful.

D.C-M (Mrs)

Candida Diet Adjusted For Cancer

Yeast associated foods to be avoided.

YEAST, BARLEY, MALT, ALCOHOL, VINEGAR, MUSHROOMS, MARMITE(YEAST EXTRACTS), SUGAR, HONEY, FRUIT & FRUIT JUICES, MOLASSES, FRUIT SUGAR, TURNIP, SWEDE, PARSNIP, BEETROOT, COOKED CARROT, GOLDEN WONDER OR FLAVOURED CRISPS, JACKET POTATO, PLAIN CRISPS, SHREDDED WHEAT, CORN FLAKES, NUTS, (UNLESS FRESHLY SHELLED), CUCUMBER, COURGETTE, MARROW, AVOCADO, SWEETCORN, WHOLE GRAINS - THESE HARBOUR PESTICIDES AND MOULDS (Even when organic they harbour moulds in storage), WATERCRESS (absorbs nitrates), COMMERCIALLY SPRAYED LETTUCE, CUCUMBER SKIN, POTATO SKIN, OUTER LEAVES OF COMMERCIALLY GROWN VEGETABLES, CHERRIES (unless organic), STRAWBERRIES (high level of histamine), SOYA SAUCE (process aids fermentation).

Permitted foods

Use first pressed, cold pressed extra virgin olive oil (not too hot when cooking to avoid free radicals). Use organic vegetables wherever possible. Chinese leaves are a safe salad alternative and Portuguese water cress. DO WASH EVERYTHING VERY WELL. Use Malvern, Evian, Volvic, Buxton, or Monastiere water etc. Use carbonated spring water or soda water for social drinking, not daily use. Use soda bread — read labels on commercial soda bread! Use organic white flour — it is a scone mix recipe, without sugar and with permitted margarine. Use corn flour and Kallo (yeast free stock cubes) for gravies. Use tea – preferably good leaf tea – Darjeeling, Assam, Luaka, or Sencha green tea (do not use tea bags – dioxins). Use raw apple, pear and banana, (one or two pieces of fruit daily - not cooked). Use unsorbated prunes, and Smiths plain crisps, For margarine use Tomor, Granovita, Pure or Granose. – make sure they are non-hydrogenated.

Use raw carrot – not cooked as it reverts to high sugar level, potato – no skin unless it is organic -, green vegetables – organic where possible and tomato (occasionally but not cooked). Use eggs (organic and wash the shells well before using), organic soya milk (unsweetened), Organic lentils (wash well before cooking). Sprout your own alfalfa, mung, and aduki beans etc.

Use white organic pasta and soya TVP (organic).

Recommended tooth pastes are: minty toothpaste or herbal toothpaste (without fluoride).

Micro-wave cooking can cause cancer and arthritis by altering the blood platelets – DO NOT USE!

READ ALL INGREDIENTS ON CONTAINERS. FOODS WITH A LONG SHELF LIFE AS THEY ALMOST ALWAYS CONTAIN PRESERVATIVES - EVEN WHEN NOT MENTIONED ON THE WRAPPER.

What next?

Once you have familiarised yourself with the banned and permitted ingredients and you are sure you have the right ingredients in stock then you are free to proceed with the Cancer/Candida diet; basically eliminating yeast, sugar, dairy products, additives and preservatives. You really must be careful!

I will give you an example of just how careful you have to be even though it still pains me to this day to think of this patient. She came to me with her husband. When she climbed the stairs to my surgery I could hear laboured breathing and, as I went to the door, I saw this lady just making the top step, pale with exhaustion and with a very swollen tummy.

My immediate thought was that I was going to deal with a pregnant asthmatic. When she had gathered her breath, I asked her, "What is the problem"? She replied, "I would like you to save my life please, I have been given three months to live; I have bowel cancer which has spread to the lungs and liver". I replied, as I always did in these cases, "I cannot guarantee to save your life but what I can assure you is that I should be able to improve the quality of your life and, as with many cases of cancer before you, when it comes, the quality of death". "Anything to improve my quality of life would be marvellous, thank you", she replied.

I then went on to do the allergy test and to explain how the pancreas works and how it malfunctions and how careful she would need to be from now on. She and her husband left with smiles on their faces and hope in their eyes. I am sorry but I do not agree with anyone having the right to tell a patient, "You are going to die" - it is what I call the witch doctor theory. It can only lead to doom and gloom.

Three weeks later this lady rang and asked me if she could go on holiday to Clovelly. Now, if any of you know Clovelly, you will know it is incredibly steep. I cautioned her and asked her to let me know how she got on. She did and I was thrilled to hear her tell me she had actually climbed Clovelly steps and was not breathless at the top and she was feeling wonderful; also that her stomach was going down.

I saw this lady on average every six weeks but kept in touch every week. Six weeks later she returned to the hospital for check up. The scan showed that the tumour, which was the size of an Ogan melon, had shrunk to the size of a golf ball — wonderful news! Three months later it had shrunk to the size of a pea, nine months later there was no sign of a tumour and a liver biopsy showed no sign of cancer cells.

This lady came to see me in March — so, you can work it out yourself, we had reached this stage just before Christmas. She sat in my surgery telling me how wonderful she felt and how I had saved her life. So far - so good. She then asked what turned out to be a fatal question," Can I have a treat for Christmas please?" I had been slowly reducing the medication and all seemed well, so why not? I said, "Yes, you can have a small piece of cake or Christmas pudding but you are to ring me immediately there appears to be a problem; yeast cells! cancer cells multiply 10 to a factor of 7 in 24 hours." Yes, that was fine.

I had my usual three days off over Christmas and, when we re-opened, the first call was from this lady's husband. "I am extremely sorry to tell you that my wife died in hospital last night. She had the Christmas cake and a few hours afterwards her tummy started to ache and swell. I asked her to ring you but she was adamant that you were not to be disturbed over Christmas. By night time she was in agony so I called the doctor. He gave her morphine and rushed her in to hospital. She passed away on Boxing Day night". He went on to thank me for everything I had done and to have achieved so much and given her back the joy of living.

It was at that moment that I realised that even as a caring practitioner there are times when you have to be cruel to be kind. When she asked if she could have a treat I should have said, "No." and I assure you that I have not made that concession again. Once you are on the candida/cancer diet, which is not difficult, then you keep to it. I have a colleague who is a Herbalist/Immunologist in Bexhill on-Sea and his treatment is almost identical to mine working on the same hypothesis. The following is just one of his many successes.

Templestowe
Victoria
Australia
D.O.B. 11-10-29
Nora suffered from a massive tumour in the uterus. She underwent a radical hysterectomy on 14th February 2001. The main part of the tumour was removed but the doctors said that the tumour had been attached to the bladder and the bowel and they had not got all of it. She suffered with constipation alternating with diarrhoea. She was unable to eat, as she was constantly nauseous. She could only walk with the aid of a wheeled walking trolley and then only for a few yards.

The doctors recommended chemotherapy. Nora heard of the wonderful results Gerald Green had been achieving with the use of wormwood (artemesia absinthium) and an anti-candida diet. As Nora was in hospital and very ill at that time, she asked her brother Bryan to contact Gerald. We were all very impressed and excited so Nora decided to embark on this treatment. She informed the doctors that she did not want to have chemotherapy. They accepted this without pressure. One of the doctors involved with her later told me that the reason for the lack of pressure was because they did not believe it (chemotherapy) would do any good but they had to offer it.

She commenced the diet immediately. (Food had to be smuggled in to the hospital, as naturally the food there was mainly unsuitable). She commenced taking the wormwood capsules on 1st March 2001. She was released from hospital on the 8th March 2001.It was necessary to take her out to the car in a wheelchair. She was unable to walk unaided, to shower herself or go unaided to the toilet. At first she was able to only eat very small meals. So she had lots of them. Essentially she grazed — always within the boundaries of the diet, exactly as instructed by Gerald, and of course she was taking the wormwood as instructed.

The progress was amazing. Each day she became stronger; each day she was able to eat more. As instructed by Gerald, she supple-

mented her diet with Echinacea and Astragalus. She was concerned about the number of bowel motions she was having — about six per day - but, as they were normal motions, Gerald assured her that this was the body's way of dealing with eliminating the toxins from the cancer.

Three weeks after commencement of the full treatment Nora was able to climb the eight stairs to come up to the dining room for her meals. She was showering herself, washing her hair, making her own bed and even helping to dry the dishes. Wonderful progress! Her appetite had increased to the stage that she was eating as much as her brother Bryan, who is a very hearty eater. Her complexion had by then lost that grey pallor and returned to her normal quite rosy colour. Bowel motions had reduced to four per day. Her weight had stabilised. She had not actually gained weight at that stage but then the anti-candida diet is hardly a 'fat gaining' diet. She then returned to live in the country with friends. She still rigidly maintained the diet. She has continued to gain strength and energy.

By the time she returned to the hospital's outpatient clinic in April for her post operative check she was walking two kilometres per day. The doctor was astounded at her progress but did not ask how or why? It has been a most remarkable experience to witness Nora's recovery.

We are all very mindful of Gerald's warning that we should regard this as remission. Nora is determined to maintain this unique treatment for the rest of her life. It is impossible to thank Gerald Green adequately for his quite remarkable work in this field and for his accessibility treatment receives the mainstream acceptance it deserves. Margaret Wheeler

(Nora's sister-in-law)

To traditional oncology the tumour is the cancer. Thus, when a tumour is removed or burned away, the patient receives an "all clear" with of course traditional reservations. The problem is, according to Krebs and Beard, the tumour is not the cause of the cancer, merely the symptom of it. If you remove the tumour – what about the proposed root cause of the cancer? Is it nutritional deficiency? Is it food sensitivity! allergens? Did the doctors dislodge cancer cells that later migrate to metastasise (spread) at other locations? How will these be killed if the root cause of the cancer is not addressed? Very commonly, as we know, secondary cancers flare up and are impossible to defeat.

So what approach would I recommend? Find a good Clinical Ecologist and determine your sensitivities; go on to the detoxification diet and take 1 teaspoon colloidal silver morning and night (from Argyll Herbs Tel:0845 8630679), Bioacidophilus powder and HEP 194(from Biocare Tel: 0121 433 3727) one of each morning and night. Within three weeks you should be feeling much better. Then commence the candida diet properly taking Wormwood *(artemesia absinthium)* as follows:

Day 1 Take 1 wormwood. cap before supper (with water)
Day 2 Take 1 cap before supper
Day 3 Take 2 caps before supper
Day 4 Take 2 caps before supper

Continue increasing in this manner until day 14 when you should be up to 7 caps. You then do 2 more days at 7 caps before supper. Then without fail, set a day aside, once a week you take 7 caps. This is for the rest of your life. Get used to it.

Black walnut hull capsules available from Topfit 01275340042/08003166714

Day 1	1 capsule
Day 2	1 capsule
Day 3	1 capsule
Day4	1 capsule
Day 5	1 capsule

Day 6 through to Day 18 Take 2 capsules and then on a maintenance dosage until candida is a distant memory – once a week maintenance programme 2 Walnut

Cloves

Day 1 Take one cap 3 times daily before meals.
Day 2 Take 2 caps 3 times daily before meals.
Day 3/4/5/6/7/8/9/10 Take 3 caps 3 times daily. After day 19 take 3 caps on same day as the other two.

I usually ask my patients to continue with an Oregano complex from Biocare as well as the aforementioned. Take one daily for at least three months. Magnesium ascorbate capsules 500mgs - take 6 daily for a month; then reduce to four. From the local health shop obtain Saw Palmetto and pumpkin seeds. Put enough pumpkin seeds to cover a 5Op piece in the palm of the hand, and then chew those thoroughly twice daily. This should reduce any inflammation and the adverse symptoms very quickly.

Prostate cancer

Let me tell you how careful you have to be. My father-in-law was diagnosed with prostate cancer that had spread to his bones, lungs, liver and kidneys. He was given three months to live at 84 years of age. He came to live with us and quite naturally we put him on a cancer control diet immediately. One of the first things we noticed, as his bedroom was next to ours, was the frequency of his visits to the toilet so we counted and were astonished to count 17 visits in 24 hours. Needless to say this was a great puzzlement to Rosemarie and myself. What was different? Then it dawned on us; as he was drinking copious amounts of tea all day and evening, could it be that the tea bags he had brought with him were the culprit? Could it be the dioxins? We changed him to a decent tea and used an infuser. The difference within three days was astounding - down to three times a night! From the local health shop obtain Saw Palmetto and pumpkin seeds. Put enough pumpkin seeds to cover a 5Op piece in the palm of the hand, and then chew those thoroughly twice daily. This should reduce any inflammation and the adverse symptoms very quickly.

Taunton
Somerset
March 2003
Dear Gwynne,
Just over a year ago I experienced one of the worst moments of my life. I sat in the hospital being told that my dear husband Tony was suffering from prostate cancer. My world fell apart. Cancer - a word that instilled total panic in me. We were told he had three choices, radical surgery (from which there would be awful side effects), or radiation therapy — ditto, or take no action and "wait and see".

The cancer was early and not very aggressive but my immediate thought was Get rid of it! It isn't that easy as you know, even the most radical cancer treatment carries NO guarantees.

Tony decided, being braver than me, that he would "wait and see' with no conventional treatment, knowing that there was another alternative with your advice.

One of the luckiest things that happened to me that year was that you, dear Gwynne, had become a regular on my TV show, and so of course I came to you and Rosemarie for help.

The first thing you did was to reduce, in my mind, the Big "C" to a small 'c ". You diminished the fear You tested Tony and recommended an anti-cancer diet. Prostate cancer as some might not know is detected by testing the blood for Prostate Specific Antigen levels (since proven to be highly inaccurate).

Here in the UK the borderline is 4. Anything over that is suspect Tony's was 4.2 when the diagnosis was made. In the USA the cut off point is 2.5.

A year later, after following the diet (which made us much healthier in many ways), Tony's PSA count, having gone from 4.2 to 3.6 to 2.6 to 2.4, is now below even the cautious USA figure. The hospital has discharged him with the proviso that he has a regular PSA check with the local GP

Gwynne and Rosemarie, it's hard to put into words how I feel about the two of you, I couldn't have survived if something had taken my Tony from me.

You didn't just save him - you saved me too.

Love

Jenny S.

Prostate cancer, or adenocarcinoma as it is called in most cases, is now the most common cancer in men in the UK. In a few years it will have overtaken lung and breast cancer and yet research is still grossly under-funded. The prostate is a gland situated between the pubic bone and the rectum and around the urethra (the tube passing from the bladder to the penis). Its function is connected with the whole urinary reproductive system.

This is again my hypothesis, we are talking about a gland — the largest gland/organ in the body is the pancreas — which, as we have said before, is responsible for producing a healthy cellular structure. If it malfunctions then glandular problems will ensue!

What are the symptoms

Difficulty or pain when passing urine.

The need to urinate more often.

Broken sleep by the need to pass urine. A long waiting period before urine flows.

The feeling that the bladder has not emptied completely.

Men are usually very slow in taking notice of symptoms and then of course when they do — it is too late! Please do not wait until it is too late — if you experience any of these symptoms go to your doctor and he will check for enlarged prostate.

Remember that a large proportion of enlarged prostate problems are non-malignant (Benign Prostatic Hyperplasia). Go to the local health shop, get some Saw Palmetto and start taking the pumpkin seeds; this will at least make sure the inflammation is reduced. Consult a qualified Clinical Ecologist and, if necessary, commence the elimination diet and the herbal parasite programme. Always remember prevention is better than cure. You can take charge of your health!

Chapter 14

Liver Problems

ANTI-FAT NUTRIENT LIPOGENESIS INHIBITORS (Inhibitors of Fat Production and Storage)

In Depth

What Are They?

Inhibitors of lipogenesis are substances which slow the production of fats from the metabolism of carbohydrates and proteins. This means inhibiting, for instance, the synthesis of triglyceridcs and/or cholesterol, Some known drugs, such as Triton, inhibit lipogenesis, but these drugs typically have side effects and they rapidly lose effectiveness with continued use. Fortunately, safe and effective natural alternatives are now being discovered. One such natural altcrnative is -hvdroxycitrjc acid, which is also called hydroxycitrate or HCA. HCA is extracted primarily from the dried pericarp (rind) of the fruit of *Garcinia cambogia.* a native plant of South Asia popularly used in cooking. including the preparation of curries. Aside from food preparation, *G. cambogia* is used as *a preservative,* as a purgative for the treatment of intestinal worms and parasites, and for bilious digestive conditions.' Traditionally, Garcinia cambogia. is said to aid the digestion and to make meals more "filling."

Anti-Fat Nutrient	Hydroxycitric Acid (HCA)
Fat Burning Function	Decreases fat production and storage.
Suggested Dose	1500 mg to several grams in divided doses with meals.

ANTI-FAT NUTRIENTS

How HCA Blocks Fat

HCA is remarkable for its ability to reduce [he body's own synthesis of fats. During the normal metabolism of meals, carbohydrate calories which are neither used immediately for energy nor stored as glycogen are converted into fats in the liver by the enzyme *ATP-citrate* Lyase.HCA inhibits this enzyme, and by doing so **it** also reduces the formation of acetyl Coenzyme A, a biochemical which plays a key role in carbohydrate and fat metabolism. As a result, the production of low density lipoprotein (LDL) and triglycerides is inhibited. The net effect is that that production and storage is reduced. The appetite is controlled, food consumption is cut and thermogenesis may be enhanced".

HCA is a substance which has been studied extensively for a period of more than two decades. Numerous animal trials conducted at major universities and described in peer-reviewed journals have demonstrated both the safety and the efficacy of HCA in inhibiting the production of fats from carbohydrate calories. The results of these trials have been so impressive that one of the world's largest pharmaceutical firms, Hoffman La Roche, not only sponsored much of the work, but also has sought synthetic versions of *HCA* which it can patent and market as diet aids. To date, no such synthetic products are available.

Because HCA has been so extensively studied, it is possible to distinguish among the various extracts available on the market. Quality control is of major importance since the desired effect is dosage-dependent. As it turns out, it is quite difficult to establish the exact amount of HCA present in an extract. Many companies which claim to have a concentration of 50% HCA actually have mistakenly counted tartaric, citric and other organic acids present in the rind as part of the HCA content. Also important is the form of HCA used. In animal trials the lactone form HCA has proven less effective than the salt form. According to data from

Hoffman- La Roche, the rate of conversion of free HCA in solution into its lactone is approximately 10% per week at low room temperature.

The Liver Cleanse

As you will have read by now, the subject of detoxification comes up continuously. The major detoxifying organ is the liver. It is often the case that the liver malfunctions and lays down excess fats (Lipogenesis). One way of reducing the laying down of fats, and preventing high cholesterol is to take a supplement from Biocare called Garcina Cambogia. In this way and with an allergy free diet, the laying down of LDL (Low density lipoprotein) and triglycerides is avoided. Where there has been an allergy/food sensitivity problem for some time the liver inevitably goes into overload and this also affects the gall bladder. Medically the answer to this is invariably the operation to remove the gall bladder. Does this solve the problem? You have guessed the answer already - NO! I do not even need to tell you why now do I? First, you must remove the cause!

In dealing with many cancer cases, the inevitable breakdown of the immune system, the toxic overload of the liver and other organs, once the candida diet and the herbal parasite programme had transpired, and the patient was feeling better, I found it almost a must to carry out the liver cleanse programme. Rosemarie and I do it twice a year as a matter of course, and I can assure you it is not difficult or painful. The following are excerpts from the *Cure for All Diseases* by Hulda Regehr Clark, PhD.ND. who I have mentioned before.

Whilst most authors reserve the right to quotation Dr Clark gives her full permission to do so. The next sentence is of paramount importance and is therefore highlighted -

Cleaning the liver bile ducts is the most powerful procedure that you can do to improve your body's health. **BUT IT SHOULD NOT BE DONE BEFORE THE PARASITE**

PROGRAMME, and for best results should follow the kidney cleanse. I am not dictating the need for the kidney cleanse but you **MUST** carry out the herbal parasite programme **FIRST** before the liver cleanse.

We have found that the best organic Epsom Salts can be. obtained from Self Health Enterprises address at rear of book.

Liver Cleanse Procedure

Ingredients

Epsom Salts 4 tablespoons

Olive Oil half cup of **light** olive oil

Fresh pink grapefruit 1 large or 2 small. Enough to squeeze 2/3 to 3/4 cup juice.

Ornithine 4 to 8 to be sure you can sleep. It can improve sleep.

Large plastic straw

Pint jar with lid

Black walnut capsules 4 to kill parasites coming from the liver.

Choose a day like a Saturday or Sunday for the cleanse since you will be able to rest the next day.

Take no medicines, vitamins or pills that you can do without, they could prevent success. **Stop the parasite programme the day before**.

Eat a **no fat** breakfast and lunch.

2.00 p.m. Do not eat or drink after 2 o'clock. Do not break this rule or you could feel quite ill later. Get your Epsom salts ready. Mix 4 tablespoons in 3 cups of water and pour this into a jar. This makes four *servings ,three quarters of a* cup each. Set the jar in the refrigerator to get it ice cold. (This is for convenience and taste only).Add a little Vit C powder to improve the taste if desired.

6.00 pm. Drink one serving (3/4 cup) of the ice cold Epsom Salts. Take the olive oil and grapefruit out to warm up.

8.00 **pm.** Repeat by drinking another 3/4 cup of Epsom Salts You haven't eaten since two o'clock, but you won't feel hungry. **Get your bed - time chores done. The timing is critical to**

success.

9.45pm Pour one 1/2 cup measure of olive oil into the pint jar. Squeeze the grapefruit by hand into the measuring cup. Remove the pulp with a fork. You should have at least 1/2 a cup full, more (up to 3/4 of a cup) is best. You may top it up with quality soda water. Add this to the olive oil. Add Black Walnut Hull. Close the jar tightly with the lid and shake hard until watery (only fresh grapefruit juice will do this).

Now visit the bathroom one or more times, even if it makes you later for your ten o'clock drink. Don't be more than fifteen minutes late. You will get fewer stones.

10.00 pm. Drink the potion you have mixed. Take 4 Ornithine tablets if you feel you will not sleep. We have not needed them. Drinking through a large plastic straw helps to get it down more easily. Take it to your bedside and standing up drink it within five minutes, the elderly may take as long as fifteen minutes. We have never had a moments problem with this, and in fact enjoy the drink.

Lie down immediately. You might fail to get any stones out if you don't. The sooner you lie down the more stones you will get out. Be ready for bed ahead of time. Lie down with your head high up on the pillow. Try to think of what is happening to the liver. Try to keep perfectly still for at least 20 minutes. You may feel a trail of stones travelling along the bile duct like marbles. There is no pain because the bile duct valves are open. Thank you Epsom Salts. Go to sleep, you may fail to get stones out if you don't.

Next morning, upon wakening, take your third dose of Epsom Salts. If you have indigestion or nausea wait until it is gone before drinking the Epsom Salts. You may go back to bed.

Don't take this potion before 6 am.

Two hours later take your fourth dose of Epsom Salts. You may go back to bed again. After two more hours you may eat. Start with fruit juice. Half an hour later eat some fruit. One hour later you may eat ordinary food, but keep it light.

Expect diarrhoea in the morning. Use a torch to look for gallstones in the toilet within the bowel movement. Look for the green kind since this is proof that they are genuine gallstones, not food residue. Only bile from the liver is pea green. The bowel movement sinks but the gallstones float because of the cholesterol inside. Count them all roughly, whether tan or green. You will need to total 2,000 stones before the liver is clean enough to rid you of allergies or bursitis or upper back pains permanently. The first cleanse may rid you of them for a few days, but as the stones from the rear travel forward they give the same symptoms again. You may repeat cleanses at two weekly intervals. Never cleanse when you are ill.

Sometimes the bile ducts are full of cholesterol crystals that did not form into round stones. They appear as 'chaff' floating on top of the toilet bowl water. It may be tan coloured, harbouring millions of tiny white crystals. Cleansing the chaff is as important as purging stones.

How safe is the liver cleanse? In my experience it is ***very safe.*** Apart from the odd patient who has experienced nausea and unable to go through to 6am there have been no reports of back problems at all. Certainly I have not had any, other than the obvious discomfort of spending considerable time in the

toilet. It certainly lowers the cholesterol levels. It is possible that you may feel slightly under the weather for a day or two afterwards, this soon *settles.*

I am going to repeat, for obvious reasons -**You must complete the herbal parasite programme first.**

Congratulations!

You have now removed your gallstones without surgery. Dr Clark likes to think she has the perfect recipe, but she certainly takes no credit for the origin, it was conceived hundreds of years ago. Thank you herbalists!

It is only right that I should tell you of a personal involvement with the liver cleanse. My dear wife Rosemarie had not changed her diet for years, other than to become a vegetarian, slowly but surely weight increased month by month, from eight and a half to nine stone to an ever increasing twelve and a half stone. From a size 8 / 10 to a size 14. Naturally we tried to think of every possibility, and like the plumber who never mends a tap at home, I probably did not give the matter as much attention as I should have done. Until one day a little glimmer of daylight peeped through the fog, we were vegetarian, we consumed olive oil every day, could it be Lipogenesis (the liver not coping with fats?), we tested and sure enough she failed. We changed to flax oil, she lost a few pounds which was good. At least she had stopped gaining. Then we considered the liver cleanse. We did exactly as Dr Clark advised us and sure enough there was a lot of 'chaff' the first time. The second time there were definitely a few small stones for both of us. They slowly increased with each cleanse to the size of peas, but then after nine liver cleanse in 12 months I produced a stone the size of a plum, amazing!!I was then, over the next year or so, able to see a transformation take place. Without changing her diet the weight started to drop off, on average 1oz per day . Rosemarie is now back to a size 8/10 and much healthier. I have never been overweight so things have not changed much for me, but I feel a lot healthier.

This procedure contradicts many medical viewpoints. Gallstones are thought to be formed in the gallbladder, not the liver. They are thought to be few, not thousands. They are not linked to pain other than gall bladder attacks. It is easy to understand why this is believed: by the time you have acute pain attacks some stones in the gall bladder are big enough and calcified enough to show up on X-Ray, and have caused inflammation there. When the gallbladder is removed the pain attacks stop. But the problem has not. Why were they there in the first place? Find the causatory 'triggers' first. The liver works very hard, why not give it a hand?

You can take charge of your health! After several liver cleanses I was proud to produce nine stones the size of a large pea, but Rosemarie produced a marble sized stone in a jar – one of 26 she had produced of this size. Finally after nine liver cleanses we produced a clear one which is when you can leave a 6 month gap. My grand finale was producing a stone the size of a greengage plum!

Xandria Williams
M.Sc., D.I.C., A.R.C.S., ND., D.B.M., M.R.N.
Naturopath, Nutritionist, Herbalist, Homeopath, Reflexologist, Psychotherapist, NLP, Reiki
Liver Detoxification:

One huge step closer to better health

by Xandria Williams

I have always loved chemistry. When I first graduated from Imperial College in London it was a toss-up between biochemistry and geochemistry. Initially I opted for the latter and worked in mineral exploration. This was at an exciting time, it was a new field, mineral exploration was going apace and I could do all the applied research I liked. It also meant I travelled the world —. mostly the southern hemisphere. However, I soon came to see the 'other side' of this research, the damage that mining was doing to the earth and the way companies used some of the results.

Personally, I had started to take an interest in 'health foods'. As a chemist, it seemed patently obvious to me that the biochemical quality and composition of a person's diet was going to have a direct impact on the structure and function of their body. It made no sense to me that ill health was being treated with compounds that had no normal function in the body, in which the body was not deficient, and which were chemical toxins with lots of nasty side effects.

I had also started to take an interest in the concept of humans as spiritual beings and came to believe that if you could help people to improve the health of their physical body then their spirit could function a lot more effectively and smoothly. This, I felt, would be something that was really worth doing and would be an exciting thing to do. This was many years ago and long before any significant training courses were available, so I began to study on my own to expand my knowledge. As a result of this I was invited to lecture first in biochemistry and then nutrition, at Sydney's Chiropractic College. This was interesting, but when, later, the Naturopathic College asked me to do the same, I suddenly found a home for my passionate interest in studies in naturopathy, herbal medicine and homeopathy in general and began my ongoing research into the links between biochemistry, human metabolism, nutrition and health. I have been in private practice, lectured and written ever since.

It seemed clear from the start that there were several important steps to helping people to better health, and that the food and the delivery system were crucially important. The diet had to be chosen for optimum nutrition and the digestive system had to be effective in breaking down the foods. Absorption and assimilation of the essential nutrients had to be optimised, as did their metabolism once inside the body. These steps alone could have improved your health. If they did not, it was then appropriate to consider whether or not you needed remedies in the form of herbs, homeopathics, or other treatments.

After twenty years in practice I am still of the same opinion, and in particular, have come to realise just how pivotally important the liver is in this whole process. It's involved in your digestion, via the gall bladder and bile. It's involved in your absorption and in the transport of nutrients. It's also involved in the processing of your waste material and toxins, many of which it excretes back into your digestive system for expulsion from the body. The liver is a vital part of your digestive system, but it is also much more than that.

The liver has literally hundreds of roles in your body

They include energy production and protein building. They include the repackaging of fats so cholesterol can be delivered to nerve and brain cells, and the rearrangement of amino acids so you have the specific ones you need. Your liver is vital for the delivery of iron to your bone marrow for the formation of new red blood cells and is part of your immune system, your hormone balance and your ability to handle stress. A healthy liver is vital for your heart, lungs, bones, kidneys and brain, in fact for your total health.

Your liver** is **a pivotal player in dealing with toxins in the body

In addition to all that your liver is a pivotal player in dealing with toxins in your body, either breaking them down into safer substances or eliminating them from the body, either as they are, or repackaged into a safer form. If all else fails, your liver will even store toxins itself, to protect the rest of the body. However, after a while, this act of generosity leads to liver damage and the rest of your body will suffer anyway.

It was this interest in the amazing and central role that your liver plays which led me to write my latest book, the 'Liver Detox Plan'. It's about your liver in general, your body's detoxification process, and an eating plan to get you back into better health. It is so vital, in dealing with any health problem, to consider the state of a person's liver and the role it may be playing in causing that problem.

Failure of your liver to perform optimally can have profound results!

Just think what can happen if your liver fails to do its job properly. It could lead to indigestion, atherosclerosis, diabetes, hormone imbalances, PMS, period or menopausal problems or headaches and migraines. You could develop allergies, leading to a vast range of symptoms ranging from eczema to asthma, migraines to arthritis, sinusitis to hives, behavioural problems, mood swings and mental confusion. You could experience blood sugar imbalances with all the many associated problems, and hundreds of different vitamin and mineral deficiency signs. You would doubtless feel tired, for many different reasons, have *poor skin and hair health. You could be an overweight but persistent yo-yo and unsuccessful dieter, and to cap it off your risk of cancer, stroke and heart disease could be greatly increased. Just think how many of your patients this list encompasses and that will give you some idea of the huge number of them that might benefit from some liver support! I know this is true in my own practice.*

It's also worth recognising just how many nutrients your liver needs and how many herbs and other compounds can help it to do its job properly. Once I had finished writing the book, I came to the conclusion that no reader would be able, nor would they in all probability, have the commitment, to go out and buy everything that had been mentioned in it. This led me to put a formulation together that contained all these substances. Furthermore, by the time I had done that I realised there were only one or two of the essential nutrients that were not included, so I decided I would include those as well. Thus it could become a multi vitamin and mineral supplement for general use but with the added advantage that it was heavily weighted towards liver support and detoxification. This is almost an essential combination for people living in our highly polluted world of inadequate diet and poor nutrition.

Detoxification problems — the silent cause

Detoxification problems may be the silent cause behind almost any symptom or health problem you may have. That's why it's important to undergo a regular detoxification programme, especially after periods of over indulgence, such as Christmas and New Year.

Prevention is better than cure

Detoxification gives your liver a period in which it can "catch up" on itself, and get rid of all the nasties it has been storing around the body. This helps to leave you feeling cleansed, revived and thoroughly rejuvenated, not to mention helping to protect against future illness. It is, after all, much easier to prevent problems, than to solve them, and once you've convinced your patients of this, they will be ***one huge step closer to better health!***

Kind regards, and a happy and healthy New Year

Xandria Williams

M.Sc., D.I.C., A.R.C.S., N.D., D.B.M., M.R.N.

Chapter 15

Arthritis

Introduction

For the last thirty five plus years I have treated patients suffering from arthritis. Initially this was by excluding certain foods such as tomato, wine, red meat and acid forming foods because these were the accepted possible causes of the condition. Success was moderate with this approach. However there was enough response to indicate that there was a link between arthritis and what we eat to pursue the subject further. Over the years, by discovering the causatory trigger and refining the way of eating to suit the individual needs of the patient, the recovery rate is nothing short of staggering.

Out of thousands of patients treated approximately 93% responded to diet and supplementation. Mention the association between arthritis and what we eat to a GP or Rheumatologist, even in this so-called enlightened age, and their response is still one of negativity - nothing is scientifically proven and is mainly apocryphal.

I have sent out hundreds of questionnaires to patients I have treated and they are poured back in. The results speak for themselves — by eliminating allergens or in some cases parasitic involvement — the arthritic condition is ameliorated. Out of every hundred responses ninety-three reported either complete elimination of the condition or, at least, elimination of swelling and reduction in pain levels, without the use of drugs. I have read many books on arthritis and will always be grateful to the authors for they were the pioneers that inspired me to persevere and perfect the procedures I use to such effect to this day. To these authors I owe gratitude and thanks: - Giraud Campbell,

Dan D. Alexander, Patricia Byrivers, Jan de Vries, Patrick Holford, John Croft, Malcolm Jayson, Allan St.J.Dixon and M. Hills.

As you will read it is not easy, and if you are faint hearted, and would rather pop a pill, **then please read no further**. However, if you are sick and tired of being told it is something you will have to live with for the rest of your life, and you know in your heart there must be some other way, then you will be encouraged, heartened and, I venture to say, excited by what you are about to discover on reading this book.

YOU DO NOT HAVE TO LIVE WITH ARTHRITIS

Foreword to Chapter on Arthritis
by Mike Finberg B.Pharm., M.R.Pharm. S.

Mike Finberg is a qualified pharmacist who moved to the West Country 25 years ago. Over the years he developed the first truly holistic pharmacy in England. This incorporated traditional pharmacy/full health food/whole food shop and Complimentary Health Centre with up to ten practitioners in varying therapies.

"I first heard about Gwynne Davies about twenty years ago through several of my customers who reported amazing improvement in their arthritic condition and others with elimination of crippling migraine attacks. I invited him to speak at our Centre - he attracted a huge crowd who listened eagerly to every word. I visited him as a patient more out of interest than need and, whilst waiting for my appointment, I noticed three or four large albums on a table. I was amazed to find them filled with unsolicited letters from grateful patients mainly to say their lives had been changed as they no longer suffered from migraines or the crippling torture of arthritis. I had worked as a medical representative for many years and never came across one, let alone an album of grateful letters. At my appointment I learnt I had a problem with butter and tomatoes amongst others. Unfortunately, as I did not at

that time have a bad arthritic problem, I ignored this preventative advice, hence six months ago I had a hip replacement, whereas Gwynne still plays golf and has not needed one. (author's note – 2004)

I have seen so many of my customers who are also patients of Mr Davies who have improved beyond their wildest dreams - but it is those that keep religiously to their new way of eating that get better. Do not forget - it is your diet for life and if you keep to it you will get better. When I lecture on Complimentary medicine - I always point out that unlike orthodox medicine, where you go to your doctor expecting him to prescribe you a pill to cure your problems (and because all drugs have side effects, you usually end up creating more problems), with complimentary therapists you are expected to help yourself in some way. With Gwynne Davies this involves excluding blacklisted foods. You are then in charge - it is up to you - you can and will get better.

I was very fortunate to meet a lovely customer who, because she was so badly arthritic, was finding her work as a probation officer almost impossible to do. I guided her to Gwynne Davies and you can read her stirring story in the book. I visited her as a client this week. She is a qualified Aromatherapist, Reflexologist, Bowtech practitioner and Remedial Masseuse - and she is brilliant. Follow her lead - take control of your life, get well, you can do it. Good luck and God Bless, and thanks Gwynne for helping to bring back health and happiness to so many people's lives.

M. FINBERG. M.R.Pharm.S"

Lighten Our Arthritic Darkness

This was the title of my second book and now adapted and updated to meet the needs of 2010. This book is now out of print.

Welcome to a world of enlightenment. I have suffered with rheumatoid arthritis and therefore know the nagging, gnawing pain, almost like a deep-seated toothache, that can keep you awake for hours at night. At times necessitating heaving yourself out of bed and walking around to loosen up, going downstairs so as not to disturb your partner, making a cup of tea, switching on the television, anything to try and obliterate the pain during the hours of darkness. After treating the condition for thirty five years plus I can tell you here and now, **YOU DO NOT HAVE TO SUFFER ARTHRITIS**!

This is no fairy tale - I am not living in cloud cuckoo land. Providing you are willing to find out what your allergens are and eliminate certain foods you will almost certainly recover. If you have had a long-term medical drug treatment, particularly gold, which is the last resort left to Rheumatologists, that alters the blood platelets irrevocably, then it may take considerably longer to obtain relief. Even in these circumstances you will find a better quality of life immediately and you will be able to look forward to recovery and repair, rather than deterioration.

I am sick and tired of hearing television and radio presenters talking about arthritis being incurable. Saying that you must learn to live with it. **Rubbish!!** If in all the years I have been practicing I had only helped a handful of patients to recover from this dreadful condition then 'they" could be right. But I am not talking about a handful, I am talking about thousands. All seen on more than one occasion and each of these cases has reported back on their condition - fulfilling the essential criteria. Many over a period of years, with no sign of a recurrence of symptoms. Doctors often say that the condition is in remission, this is when symptoms subside but flare again at some later date. The only time my patients suffer from a 'flare' is when for one reason or another they have strayed from their diet. So gird up your loins, deep breath, say to yourself, **"I will do it",** and then you will find **YOU DO NOT HAVE TO LIVE WITH ARTHRITIS!!**

I do not pretend for one moment that it is easy - in most cases it certainly is not. My experience tells me that men find it much harder to keep to a diet than women. Generally speaking this is because men are invariably more sociable, and therefore find it harder to give up favourite foods, alcohol etc: The Friday or Saturday night out with the boys is not easy to forego, but there is nothing wrong with going out for the night with the boys is there? Maybe even a 7 Up or still or sparkling water is better than pain. Always check the ingredients though and that will prove how strong minded you are. I find that women generally are able to apply themselves much more assiduously and certainly maintain the strict protocol for much longer. I would say this is because they are at home, able to shop for the right foods, and spend more time on the preparation than the average male does. This is why I believe that women have such an important part to play if it is their partner that is suffering. They are able to control the dietary intake of food and drink to a greater degree, packing up lunches if necessary, and of course encouraging their partner to stick with it and not to give way to temptation. It has certainly proved in the past that if both partners go on the diet together it is most beneficial and in many cases, although the partner was not suffering, they feel enormous benefit in their general health and vitality.

This could also be a subjective judgment on my part. Over the thirty five years I have certainly seen far more women than men with the dreaded arthritic condition. Another problem that manifests itself is that most men like their alcohol and have a terrible sweet tooth. I know I have, and this is not easy to give up either. I can think of a couple of occasions where a male patient has said, " I will do everything you tell me, but I will not give up my scotch". I have to say that he got away with drinking a glass of scotch occasionally, but this only occurred with one patient and I would certainly not recommended it.

However this certainly does not apply to all of us – he was privileged to be lucky enough to escape unharmed; it is not a recommended course of action. Certainly I could not do that without suffering the next day. So, particularly in the early stages of the diet, do not be tempted to stray from the guidelines.

What is arthritis? Depending on which book you read, interpretations differ. There are many books on arthritis in circulation and each one will tell you something different with regard to recovery. Why I believe this book is so different, and should be so helpful is that it is not based on speculation, nor because it has worked for a limited number of people, but it is based on the clinical evidence of many thousands of patients over a thirty five year period.

Always being one to try and simplify things I would say it is a very painful condition affecting the bones and muscles, ligaments, tendons, discs and synovial sacs between large joints. It may be rather cynical of me to adopt this attitude, but I have been convinced for most of my time in practice that the medical profession and scientists love to give things long complicated names to totally confuse the layman. It is amazing when you listen to two Doctors or Specialists talking about your condition, it is as if they were speaking a foreign language. I hope you are the same as me and like to be told what is wrong, in good old basic English, and what you can do to correct it. **You do not have to live with it**, and in this book you will be getting advice on how to overcome it.

The two most common types of arthritis are osteo-arthritis and rheumatoid arthritis, the first affecting the bone structure and commonly referred to as wear and tear - and the second affecting the musculature and ligamenture. These are fairly straightforward. Then we get on to the more complicated conditions

Systemic Lupus Erythamatosus - a chronic inflammatory disease of connective tissue, affecting the skin and various internal organs - treatment -corticosteroids.

Lumbar Spondylitis - inflammation of the synovial joints of the backbone — treatment - non steroidal anti-inflammatory drugs.

Ankylosing Spondylitis - a rheumatic disease involving the backbone and sacroiliac joints, and sometimes causes arthritis in the shoulders and hips - treatment - analgesics.

Reiters Syndrome - a disease of men involving diarrhoea, inflammation of the urethra and conjunctiva and arthritis - treatment - steroids.

Cervical Spondylosis - degeneration of the intervertebral discs in the cervical region. Spondilosis can also occur in the thoracic or lumbar region - treatment - non steroidal anti-inflammatory drugs (N.S.A.I.D's).

Osgood Schiatters Disease - mostly affecting the young and the knee joints mainly involved.

Pagets Disease - a chronic disease of the bones, occurring in the elderly and most frequently affecting the skull, backbone, pelvis and long bones. Affected bones become thickened and severe pain ensues - treatment - anti-inflammatory drugs.

Polyarthritica Rheumatica - inflammation of many joints, - treatment - N.S.A.I.D's.

As far as I am concerned these are bone or muscular conditions that mean pain and discomfort and in some cases the distortion of joints - **and YOU DO NOT HAVE TO LIVE WITH IT!**

So, what is arthritis? Some mystery disease that affects nearly eight million people in the UK? Or is it a, mystery? As I hope to show you as we proceed through the chapter that it is not a mystery at all - I call it an allergy reaction. But what is allergy?

There have been numerous books on arthritis, written over the years, where putting the author's partner on a special diet and avoiding certain foods has eliminated the condition. Marvellous, I am not knocking that approach, it is just that I believe it is much more individualistic than that, as each person reacts in their own way. The clinical evidence I have amassed over the last thirty-five or so years, using applied kinesiology, (muscle/nerve reflex response to a substance placed under the tongue) has convinced me that there is an overall pattern observed and if we adopt that pattern initially most people will respond. Kinesiology is taught in many colleges throughout the U.K. and they all have their own way of teaching this sensitive and applied method of testing for allergens and vitamin and mineral deficiencies. Whatever method is used the results are generally good enough to determine food sensitivities and set you on the road to recovery. Remember also that the body changes once detoxification has taken place, so, if you are still having problems after a period of weeks then go back for a recheck. I have had many patients over the years that suffered with horrendous migraine headaches and when tested initially showed the typical 4C Syndrome (coffee cheese citrus chocolate) but no sensitivity to dairy products. The headaches had resolved and months later the patient is back complaining of a totally different symptom. A re-check found the patient to be totally sensitive to dairy products. A classic case of 'unmasking'. The predominant allergen manifesting themselves and sublimating the underlying and, in many cases, the primary cause of the initial symptoms.

What happens then

I hope that has helped you to understand the link between allergy and arthritis. Let me for a moment try and bring these entities together, and do not be alarmed; it is inclined to be heavy going so do not be surprised if you have to read it again to make sense of it. Remember this is my hypothesis, but one that has proved to be correct in the assessment and successful treatment of arthritics over time. As I have mentioned previously I believe the cause to be a pancreatic malfunction. The inability of the pancreas to recognise the enzymes in certain foods- 'invaders' causing a release of mast cell toxins (compartmentalised throughout the body and to which the antibodies attach) which then permeate the system insidiously as with osteo-arthritis and, in many cases, instantly with rheumatoid type reactions. In the lipase, amylase, trypsinogen phase of pancreatic function we should break down the enzymes and produce enterokinase or enteropeptinase in the duodenum, this then produces healthy cellular function. When this does not happen kinin and subsequently bradikinin are produced, a breakdown in the normal processes, and pain and discomfort ensue.

Kinin is one of a group of naturally occurring polypeptides that are powerful vasodilators, which lower blood pressure, and cause contraction of smooth muscle. The kinins (bradikinin and kallidin) are formed in the blood by the action of proteolytic enzymes (kallikreins) on certain plasma globulins (kininogens). Kinins are not normally present in the blood, but are formed under certain conditions; for example when tissue is damaged, or when there are changes in the pH and temperature of the blood. - They are thought to play a role in inflammatory response.

In his book, *Allergies - Your Hidden Enemy,* Dr Theron Randolph M.D. (the alma mater of Clinical Ecology) devotes a whole chapter to arthritis, and the association between this condition and food substances and chemical susceptibility. The first definitive work was published by Doctor Michael Zeller in 1949 and titled, *Rheumatoid Arthritis - Food Allergy as a Factor.* These men were the pioneers of clinical ecology and its use in the relief of debilitating diseases.

Since the 1920's medical practitioners have been recording individual maladaptive reactions to foods and chemicals, observed as emerging during controlled systematic test exposures.

The tests I have carried out over the past years are conclusive evidence that the pancreas, the INSTIGATORY endocrine exocrine ducts of the body, gives us the key to relieving the many debilitating conditions prevalent in society today. Arthritis in all its guises, and they are numerous, is an inflammatory condition, with the exception of osteo-arthritis which is mainly wear and tear.

At this point I would like to quote from a book that has been very important to me in understanding the psychology of disease. It is called *Brain Allergies - The Psychonutrient Connection,* Kalita and Philpott - both MD's. The following is a quote from that book. *"The 'hard way' to discover truth need not be the only one. We must always keep in mind that the greatest enemy of any science or any discovery of truth is a closed mind. Accordingly, we should seek the courage to ask impertinent questions which will shake our complacency, challenge our minds and to look deeper into the farthest reaches of the great mystery- of the human body. Then and only then will we be able to accept truth at face value".*

It is very easy to become complacent and say, "aren't I a clever lad, and why doesn't the rest of the world agree with me?" Particularly when the methodology I use proves to be so successful. Believe me I am humbled and appreciative of the guidance I have been given, and the ability to study at an age when that should be behind us. It is still encouraging when you study tomes like Brain Allergies to discover that your insistence on maintaining a simplistic and unrecognised practise has in fact been corroborated.

The inclusion of case histories is to give you, the reader, the opportunity to share with fellow sufferers what you are going through. I am sure that those of you who suffer with arthritis will identify with at least one of the cases. The first one is very typical of what does happen and how you too can help ameliorate your condition.

MrsD. T
Isle of Wight.
"It was a Wednesday afternoon middle of May 1978 when I started to feel poorly. It started with a headache at the back of my head, which eventually came up over the top and I thought I had caught a heavy cold. I went to bed early and awoke the next morning with fingers as big as sausages and very painful. On the Friday I was feeling quite poorly and in pain so my husband decided to ring a specialist for a private appointment. He said he would see me on the Saturday morning. He went into my past health history and I told him that at the age of twelve I had rheumatic fever. After an examination he referred me to the local hospital for blood tests and asked me to come back the following Wednesday for the results. We did, and my husband and I were absolutely shattered when he told us I had Rheumatoid Arthritis and would be in a wheel chair within three years. We walked away absolutely devastated but my husband Ron said to me, "if they think I am going to wheel you around in a wheel chair after the hard working life we have had they have another think coming, we are going to fight this thing".

The doctor had even told my husband we would have to sell the business because I would not be able to cope. So the fight began. I went back to my own G. P and he then told us he was putting me on Opren. My husband asked him what the side effects would be. "Oh!" he said, "not much, she may get indigestion or a rash or she won't be able to go out in the sunlight". As I had never suffered these things and I love the sun I refused to take this drug, wasn't I the lucky one!!

So, my husband decided to take me to Harley Street for a second opinion, but there I was told more or less, "hard cheese, you will have to learn to live with it". I had attended physiotherapy sessions Mon / Wed/Fri that left me in agony on Tues/Thurs/Sat/Sunday, so I decided I would not go, and by now the pain was all over my body. We had a Post Office and I found I could not count the notes very well and it was very painful to tear the stamps, but I plodded on.

Every so often I had to attend the Rheumatoid Clinic where the Specialist was very off hand and not a bit sympathetic, so one day the nurse said to me, "how are you today Mrs T?" I had to tell her that I felt very poorly, I pained everywhere and there was very little let up, and I am afraid I was a little down that day.

Oh! let me go back to the Christmas, because this is now February 1979 and we had gone to my daughter Gillian's for Christmas, and on Boxing Day she held open house for all my old friends. I was sitting on the settee and one of my friends asked Gillian where I was and Gillian told her I was on the settee, and her reply was, "not that little old lady?" Now I am anything but a little old lady but that is just what I looked like. A few days later after we got home I had a letter from that friend with a card enclosed and it said, "Doreen go and see this man, you will never regret it."

Now I will go back to my visit to the specialist. The nurse said I want you to get undressed Mrs T because he has never examined you properly. I was called in to his office feeling very poorly. He was sitting at his desk writing and did not even look up, even when I said "good morning", he just said, "what can I do for you". I told him I was feeling very poorly and his answer then sent me in to floods of tears. He said, "You are like my car standing outside. You need all new spare parts and I cannot give them to you. You seem to think you can get better on hard work and brown bread but it will not work and you have not attended physiotherapy, in fact I do not wish to see you again." I was devastated and told him that I did not wish to see him again either

When I got back to the Post Office my girls who worked for us told my husband to "go upstairs and sort me out. That was when he rang the number on the card my friend sent and made an appointment to see Gwynne Davies,

I saw Gwynne Davies in February 1979 and he informed me it was a pancreatic malfunction causing the problem and I was producing a pain transmitting hormone called kinin, this was breaking down in to bradikinins, tiny razor edged crystals and these were attacking the joints and creating the inflammation. He tested me for my allergies and told me to avoid all milk products, oranges, tomatoes, rhubarb, gooseberry, strawberry, beetroot, spinach, peppers and radish. Peel apples and wash all fruit thoroughly. He then put me on a strict arthritic diet and within three weeks I noticed a decrease in the pain and started to improve. I am now free of pain and stiffness and providing I do not stray from the straight and narrow I feel fine.

To summarise, in May 1978 1 was told I would be in a wheel chair within three years, I started the treatment with Gwynne Davies in 1979, it is now sixteen years on and I am 68 years of age, and I can give many a 40 year old a run for their money

So, you see, **YOU DO NOT HAVE TO LIVE WITH ARTHRITIS!**

It is now 2010 and this lady and her family have become dear friends, so, I see her quite regularly, and 31 years later, yes she is now 81, she is marvellous, thank you Doreen for being such a model patient.

Patients often ask me which food is the biggest culprit? As I pointed out earlier, there have been many books published on arthritis, and therefore there have been differing opinions as to the major culprits, many of these pure hypotheses. What I am trying to do in this book is to tell you what has worked so well in a clinical situation treating not a handful but thousands of patients. I have to be honest and say the biggest culprit is milk.

Living in a rural area like Taunton in Somerset, with hundreds of dairy farmers and dairy farmers' wives as patients, you can imagine that statement goes down like a lead balloon but it is a fact. Out of the thousands of arthritic patients that have consulted me over the years at least 90% are allergic to milk and associated products. Certainly where osteo arthritis is concerned milk is always the major culprit. Where rheumatoid arthritis is concerned then milk is usually the basic causatory 'trigger' but exacerbated by so called acid foods.

...n challenged on the use of the word allergy. Because ...rue immunological response it is not correct to use the ...ord allergy, we should use hypersensitivity, but we are not here to split hairs. The main thing as far as I am concerned is that patients understand that they cannot tolerate dairy products. Allergy is a word most people understand and can come to terms with. Whatever you call it - hypersensitivity or allergy - the results are the same- pain, stiffness and swelling. So in a moment let us look in more depth at milk, and the possible reasons we cannot tolerate it. I often say, "It is simple, a cow has four stomachs and we only have one, so how can we digest it. What is a cow's natural diet? It eats grass'.

Needless to say there are differing viewpoints as to why milk is so deleterious to our health generally. Certainly the Milk Marketing Board (as it used to be called) will disagree with these assumptions but one would expect them to. They are in the business of getting you, the public, to drink as much as possible to make a profit from their customers.

When you think of the millions of pounds already spent, and still being spent on advertising this product, it is not surprising the public has fallen for it.

MILK IS GOOD FOR YOU! DRINK A PINTA DAILY! YOU NEED MILK TO GET CALCIUM AND BUILD HEALTHY BONES!

What a load of nonsense that all is. Admittedly we all need calcium and other minerals to build healthy bones, nails, teeth and hair, but milk is not the way to get it. Have you ever seen a native of Africa or an Eskimo with bad nails, teeth, hair or bones? I have not, and they do not generally drink milk, unless they have been in this country for some time and have become westernised in their dietary habits. When did you last see an elephant drinking milk? I think you will agree they are strong enough.

What have we done to our milk over the years? HOMOGENISING - we are told that this is a good process and very necessary. It permits milk to stand around longer without going sour. It allows fat globules to emulsify and the cream does not separate. We do not have to go to the enormous trouble of shaking the bottle each time, very tiring. But there is a price to pay for saving our muscle strength and making fewer trips to the local shop. The process of homogenisation/pasteurisation consists of putting milk under high pressure and elevated temperatures 131-158 degrees F. It is a 'flash' process that does not remove the mutated IgFl. This changes the raw protein in milk and makes it less nutritional. It destroys an enzyme called phosphatase, which is necessary for the utilisation of calcium and phosphorous. It destroys some of the valuable B-Vitamins and some of the C vitamins. Right up until the early 1900's milk was a whole food. It was not skimmed, boiled, powdered, condensed, pasteurised or homogenised. I know, yes, you are quite right, occasionally it was certified. But what did that mean? It was a means of ensuring that through controlled feeding conditions, the milk was nutritious, fresh, and hygienic and TB tested. BUT IT WAS NOT PROCESSED!

You do not need to be an Einstein to see that the many hundreds of changes that have taken place with the production, feeding, and de-naturisation of pastureland, the precious 'balance of nature' has been destroyed,(nitrites and nitrates) and the consequences of absorption within our own bodies affected. Ask any opera singer why they do not ingest milk products?

There was a time when I thought that raw milk was the best thing for patients. In other words straight from the cow, no homogenisation or pasteurisation. In the early days of testing patients on raw milk many tolerated it quite happily, however this view has changed over the years for many reasons. Again it is only my viewpoint but I do firmly believe that the treatment of the grasslands, the use of antibiotics in foodstuffs for calves, and the increased weakening of their immune systems have created the situation we are now faced with where 95-98% of arthritics tested are allergic to it. Thankfully there is an alternative, goats or sheep's milk, and let us put this bogey to bed about these alternative milks not being so good for you. From a nutritional point of view, ewe's milk is the most concentrated milk food. Typical differences in the energy value of the three milks are expressed here in kilocalories (kcal) as well as in the modern terminology of kilojoules (kJ)

1 calorie=184 joules.

	Kcl	kjoule
Sheep	102	426
Goat	71	296
Cow	65	272

Olive Mills - Thorsons 1982, took these figures from *Practical Sheep Dairying*. Weight or volume tables can be found on page 158/159 in the above-mentioned book.

Another good reference, for anyone interested in following tables of comparisons, is *Health Hazards* of *Milk* by D. L. J. Freed, Bailliere Tindall, 1984. Professor Freed is Lecturer in Immunology, Department of Bacteriology and Virology, University of Manchester. I can assure you that the difference in calcium levels between them is so little it is not worth considering.

You will appreciate of course that goats and sheep's milks are full fat and, in the early stages of the diet when the major detoxification is taking place and the poor old liver has to work overtime, I recommend that you dilute them with 50% water. This at least gives the liver a chance to decongest and absorb proteins more readily and the fats of course. In the leaflet I give to patients outlining the dangers of milk consumption, the following are pertinent.

The milk of any species was designed for one purpose only to feed its young. Human beings are the only creatures on this earth that drink the milk designed for another species and we continue to do so all our adult lives, never weaning ourselves off it. Can you imagine a calf, kid, or lamb trying to continue feeding from its parent? It would be kicked off and encouraged to eat grass as nature intended. What do we do to the poor old cow? We encourage it to continue pumping out milk every day of its life and for what purpose? - to feed human beings who are continually bombarded by radio, television and advertising, plus the medical profession, to drink milk because it is good for them. If you saw the state of the bone structure of some of my patients you would soon realise that it is not good for you at all and, far from feeding the bones, cow's milk actually depletes the bone structure by an autoimmune response, slowly but surely diminishing the periosteum and causing the bone to become porotic (porous).

The enzymes we need to break down and digest milk are rennin and lactase. By the age of four many of us lose the ability to digest lactose because we can no longer synthesise the digestive enzyme lactase. This lactose intolerance results in diarrhoea, flatulence and bowel or stomach cramps. Some 90% of adult Asian and black people, and 20% of Caucasian children are lactose intolerant.

The level of protein (casein) in cow's milk is 300 times higher than the protein (predominantly lactalbumin) in human breast milk, which is easily digestible by babies. Nature has designed the milk of each animal species specifically to meet the needs of its young. Casein is intended to be broken down by the four-stomach digestive system of baby cows. In human stomachs it coagulates and forms large tough, dense, difficult to digest curds, When the protein of another animal is introduced into the body, it may cause an allergic reaction (Journal of Allergy, 41: 226, 1968.) the most common symptoms of which are chronic runny nose, persistent sore throat, hoarseness, bronchitis and recurrent ear infections.

THE MUCOUS MEMBRANES LINING THE JOINTS AND LUNGS CAN BECOME SWOLLEN OR INFLAMED. CONTRIBUTING TO RHEUMATOID ARTHRITIS AND ASTHMA. Underlined to bring the point home to you.

As I have mentioned already, milk is touted as a great natural source of calcium and we are told to ingest calcium to prevent osteoporosis or thinning of the bones. In fact eating dairy products can increase the rate at which calcium is lost from the bones and so hasten osteoporosis.

As well as being high in calcium dairy products are also high protein foods. If we have too much protein in the diet from milk products or any other source such as meat, fish, or eggs, the body has to get rid of the excess. To do this the kidneys must lose calcium as they cleanse the blood of excess waste, a process known as protein induced hypercalcuria.

People in the United States and Scandinavia consume more dairy products than anywhere else in the world, yet they have the highest rate of osteoporosis; (Clin Ortho Related Res,

35,1980). This fact emphasises the threat of excessive protein in the diet and suggests that dairy products offer no protection against osteoporosis, probably due to the high content of milk. (Am J Clin Nutr, 41; 254,1985).

The body's ability to absorb and use calcium depends on the amount of phosphorous in the diet. The higher the calcium phosphorus ratio the less bone loss takes place and the stronger the skeleton, providing the intake of protein is not excessive. The foods, which contain higher calcium phosphorus ratios, are. fruit and vegetables. Low fat milk is no better for you either, remember - a little does do harm!

Low fat milk contains one per cent butter fat and the full compliment of allergy inducing milk protein!

Getting bored with all this talk of the dangers of ingesting milk? I hope not for there is more to come yet... But let us break for a moment the intensity of the subject and —'lighten your darkness' - by quoting another case history from someone who is allergic to milk.

MrsD.S.
Waterlooville, Hants.
Before I consulted Gwynne Davies my condition had deteriorated a great deal since first visiting my GP and a Rheumatologists who could offer no hope of improvement and would prescribe stronger drugs. I was sent to the local hand clinic of the local hospital that gave me hand splints to help straighten my fingers. I had reached a stage where I could not hold a newspaper without a lot of pain in my hands and forearms. I could not lift a bag of sugar, a kettle, or make the beds because I could not bear the weight on my hands I found it impossible to turn the ignition key of the car and was so tired I needed a rest every-afternoon, which was totally out of character. I seldom could take a bath because I could not get out, neither my wrists nor my knees were strong enough to lift me and I could only walk a short distance.

Within a few days of starting the treatment recommended by Gwynne Davies I lost most of the pain and, within two weeks, there was a marked improvement in my health. At the beginning I weighed about 11 stone 10 lbs. I am now 10 stone. After twenty-one months I am a different person, much more active both physically and mentally, and I play an active part in the community again.

I can now run a home, drive a car and take my dog and my grandchildren for long walks. I have taken up swimming for the first time and, as a keen horsewoman, I am considering riding again. It has been a wonderful cure, and every day I give thanks for the skills of Gwynne Davies.

So you see, **YOU DO NOT HAVE TO LIVE WITH ARTHRITIS!**

Now to return to the thorny subject of milk. Added to the list of problems already mentioned we can also add a host of unnatural ones. Cow's milk contains the accumulated pesticides that have been sprayed on to the grain to feed the cattle, and the pastureland, and the female hormones given to cows to increase milk production and body fat. Some milk has also been shown to contain trace metals- and radioactivity at levels higher than those permissible in drinking water. There is also the thorny problem – not yet resolved of GM crops being used as cattle feed.

Some 20% of milk producing cows in America are infected with leukaemia a virus, which, because the milk is pooled when collected, infects the whole milk supply. What a scenario! These cancer-inducing viruses are resistant to being killed by pasteurisation and have been recovered from supermarket supplies *(Medical World News, 16* May,1989). Can it really be coincidence that the highest rates of leukaemia are found in children aged 3 - 13 years of age who consume the most milk products and in dairy farmers who, as a profession, have the highest rates of leukaemia in any group? I think not.

I certainly do not wish to bore you with a book full of statistics. Apart from anything else they can be massaged in such a way as to show what one wishes to show. But at the same time I have to look at the clinical evidence, the proof of the pudding as it were. This speaks volumes and I hope to show this throughout the book. 95-98% of all arthritic patients I have treated, and they run into many thousands, have been allergic to cow's milk. What is even more important is that they have all reaped benefit by eliminating it from their diets. As I said earlier it is contrary to the chapter on arthritis in my first book, "Overcoming Food Allergies", Ashgrove Press, 1985. The evidence was not available or as clear-cut as it is now and, if this book is going to help those suffering from the dreaded arthritis or osteoporosis, this evidence must be made available. Times change and statistics alter.

You will hear me repeating time and time again, do not think by just eliminating milk you have solved the problem. The plain and simple fact is you have not. It is much more complicated than that. The elimination of all dairy products from ones diet is no easy matter. You will need to check labels at all times. I am asked so many times by patients, "Is it alright when I am out if I have just a little?" My reply is always the same, No; you might just as well have a bucketful! I certainly know when I have had something wrong. My hands are stiff and the skin sensitive, and my hip and knee hurt.

One lady came back for a second appointment and showed me her hands and the fingers were like small sausages. "What on earth have you been doing?" I asked. "Well I find it difficult to believe but a few nights ago I went out for a meal with friends and had some butter in a sauce, surely it cannot be that?" The answer is of course. "Yes it was just that." After ten days the toxins had cleared again and she was fine.

Milk really does lurk in the most unlikely places. Who would think that if you had a gravy made with Bovril that you were having milk? But you are, there is lactose in it. Who would think when you accepted a wine gum and ate it that you were ingesting lactic acid? But you are and it is there in the small print, and sometimes very, very small print.

Oh! I can't have butter, never mind I will have margarine. No you cannot! Many margarines contain lactic acid and whey, both milk derivatives. There are alternatives - at present they are available in health shops. I believe it will not be long before the margarine manufacturers will be producing non- hydrogenated margarines as a matter of course, if you look carefully you will see margarines in Supermarkets that do state that they are non-hydrogenated and contain no transfatty acids. Also of great importance it should state NO G.M.(Genetically modified foods. Make sure you read the small print. You will no doubt be aware from television and newspapers that a war has gone on for years with each side arguing the merits of their own product - quite understandably of course. So, which margarines can you have that are safe? WHOLE EARTH, VITAQUELLE, MUNSTERLAND and PURE, ALL OF THESE SHOULD STATE THEY ARE ORGANIC. These are all non-hydrogenated margarines, with no trans-fatty acids, much better for you, and can be used for cooking. Having said that, for pastry making when you are fit and well enough, then Munsterland from the supermarket is the one of choice. It is a German margarine.

Help! that means I cannot have cheese! Not true, you can, and what is more they are delicious. I will try and list some of the most popular ones. CHEVRES, HALUMI, EFTAKI, FETA, PECORINO, MANCHEGO, CABRALES, ROCQUEFORT plus many other goat and ewes milk cheeses. A choice selection for anyone. It is very rare these days to find a cheese with animal rennet in it. We have also found by experimentation that you can cook ordinary cheese IN THE OVEN not the grill and this is fine too. Some health shops will tell you that this is not permissible if you are allergic to dairy products because it is made with cow's milk. This is not true either. I have tested patients for a long time now and the cooked cheese in the oven appears to be perfectly safe and as yet no allergic reactions observed.

Are there alternative milks? Of course there are. Goats milk, sheep's milk, oat milk (thick and filling, check also for any reaction such as bloating,) rice milk usually sold as Rice Dream, very pleasant for cereals if allowed, and soya. I have to be honest and say that I do not like soya milk as it leaves a dry nutty taste in the mouth but hundreds of patients tell me they quite like it in preference to goats or sheep's. Also many Soya milks contain sugar and, as mentioned elsewhere this may be bad for you. We are all individuals thank goodness and all our tastes are different. What a dreary old world this would be were that not so. I have certainly found that sheep's milk does not vary very much at all in taste or texture, but goat milk does. So if you are not happy with the one you have tried, do shop around until you find one you do like. . Do not put babies on to goats or sheep's milk without advice from a practitioner. There are several organic soya milks on the market; PLAMIL, PROSOBEE ETC. Avoid UHT or Pasteurised goats or sheep's milk if possible.

DANGER! BEWARE! If you have a milk allergy; avoid the following:-LACTOSE, LACTASE, LACTIC ACID E270, CASEIN, WHEY, SKIMMED MILK.

The under mentioned products can, and frequently do, contain milk in one form or another. It will drive you mad shopping for approximately three weeks while you read all the labels, and get used to which products are safe, but you must check!

Baking Powder, Biscuits, Baker's bread (sliced packet loaves), Bavarian cream, Crème brule, panacotta, Boiled salad dressings, Bologna, Butter, Buttermilk, Butter sauces, Cakes, Chocolates, Chocolate or Cocoa drinks or mixtures, Cream, Creamed foods, Cream sauces, Cheeses, Curds, Custards, Doughnuts, Eggs scrambled, Escallop dishes, Foods prepared au gratin, Food fried in butter- Fish, Poultry, Beef, Pork, Ham, Bacon, Veal), Flour mixtures, Fritters, Gravies, Hamburgers, Hash, Turkey breast and Turkey roll, some frozen turkey, some chicken breasts, Hard sauces, Ice creams, Mashed potato, Malted milk, Ovaltine, Meat loaf, Cooked sausages, Omelettes, Oleomargarines, Pastry crust, Popcorn, Prepared food mixes for biscuits, cakes, muffins, pancake, piecrust, waffles and puddings, Rarebits, Salad dressing, Sherberts, Souffles, Some Soups, Sweets, Some low fat crisps.

This list is a guide. Manufacturers do change the contents of their products frequently, so, be on your guard and make vigilance your password. A classic example of this was several years ago when I advised patients to use 'Outline" margarine as it did not contain lactose; I then started getting phone calls from all over the country from patients complaining that many of their old symptoms had returned. When I contacted Van Den Bergh, the manufacturer, it had decided, in its wisdom, to add lactose and call it "NEW Outline". When the patients were advised of this and they removed it from their diet their symptoms soon disappeared.

You will remember earlier I mentioned pork ham, bacon and veal as being wrong to eat. This is because to this day, although not as frequently as in the past, whey is used to feed pigs, and calves to become veal, and whey is a milk by-product. However if you know a butcher that can supply non-whey fed pork then you are allowed to eat this. Do please note that because it may be stated that it is organic pork, this does not mean it is not whey fed, it invariably is. It really is amazing how many patients say, "I cannot eat pork it makes me ill. On the pages that will follow, recommending the foods to eat, you will see meat mentioned, this is an endeavour to balance out the diet as much as possible. The diet really is predominantly fruit and vegetables; and if at all possible eat organic food. If you can grow your own without the use of pesticides and sprays, then so much the better. Rare breeds' meat and poultry has to be tasted to be believed, and can be sampled by appointment at, The Bell and Bird Table, Runnington, Wellington, Somerset.01823663080 Another excellent source of organic meat which can be delivered all over the country is Riverford Organics.

When I tell you that the McGrath's meat and poultry is used in some of the top hotels in the country you will realise just how special it is. Needless to say you cannot just turn up and buy it; orders do have to be made in plenty of time. During the war, and that gives my age away, those of you who remember those days will remember how bacon used to cook, simmering away gently in the frying pan and with that special smell and the taste! What is more, when you cook organic pork the crackling actually crackles! Nowadays the bacon spatters all over the kitchen, the smell is not at all appetising and the taste is only moderately acceptable.

In a previous book I recommended the ingestion of organ meats (liver, kidneys etc) as being good for you. I no longer believe this to be true and recommend that unless things change dramatically over the next five years or so do not eat organ meats! A question I am often asked is, "How long do I have to keep to the diet?" The answer of course – forever, if you wish to stay free of swelling and pain. I have kept to it for twenty-five years now and have no intention of detracting from, it. If you were born with a pancreatic malfunction, which produces a pain transmitting hormone bradykinin, then until such times as someone gives you a replacement you keep to the straight and narrow. As I have said before, it is straight and, at times when friends and relatives are filling their faces with goodies, it is very narrow! However they are not the ones that suffer with the pain or the swelling, so you do not listen when in all sincerity they say, "Oh! go on a little can't hurt surely." But we know different don't we? I suffer from psoriasis as well as arthritis and if I detract from the straight and narrow, which thankfully does not happen deliberately or very often, then my hands become stiff and swollen and the psoriasis will appear somewhere on my body. So I learnt many years ago it just is not worth it. I am quite sure that once you have experienced the joy of moving freely again, without pain or swelling then you too will not wish to stray.

In the majority of cases the condition has not flared up overnight. It has been one of slow but sure deterioration. But some patients with rheumatoid arthritis report that they went to bed with no pain at all and, in the early hours of the morning, they were woken up with awful pains in the joints and in most cases swollen joints too. Very often there is reddening and heat can be felt emanating from a particular joint or joints. Quite sensibly the patient reports to the GP and invariably what happens? The patient is prescribed an anti-inflammatory drug, NSAID, of which more in the next chapter. A blood sample is then taken and sent to the laboratory and the results are confirmed within fourteen days. It really-is amazing how these results vary. Many are told that the result is positive and to take the NSAIDS and, if the pain gets worse, come back and have something stronger or at worst you may need operative procedures. How I wish GP's would realise that much could be done by alternative means and not to create this 'abandon hope' attitude. It is only fair to mention at this juncture that some patients with mild arthritic pain do benefit from taking NSAIDS. Others are told that the results are negative so there is nothing further that can be done.

Now let us take a few salient points from an earlier paragraph. The joint can be swollen and reddened and heat can be felt emanating from it. Certainly, in the case of hands and feet distortion of these limbs can be seen in a comparatively short space of time; this is invariably rheumatoid arthritis and is extremely painful. It really is quite amazing how many patients have related the above to me and presented with the obvious symptoms and yet they have been told the tests are negative and we do not know what the condition is, it could get worse and you will have to live with it.

I recall vividly, something like fifteen years ago; a young lady in her thirties consulted me with her husband. She came from Bridgwater and her hands were distorted and swollen. The pain was excruciating and preventing her from sleeping properly. She presented herself to her GP three times, blood samples were sent off and returned as negative, to be told by her doctor that she did not have rheumatoid arthritis.

What did she have then? Surely the doctor had been in practice long enough to recognise the condition without the need of blood tests. I informed her that I had seen enough of the condition over the years to recognise it as rheumatoid arthritis and I would be treating her as such. On testing she proved hypersensitive to, have you guessed yet? of course you have - dairy products!! There were other products, apple skin, tomato, rhubarb, gooseberry, strawberry, beetroot, spinach, peppers, and radish and, because of the rheumatoid involvement, she was told to blanch her onions and leeks, asparagus and celery. As there is an involvement with oxalic acid these foods need to be monitored very carefully. Off she went home to Bridgwater with her husband, both in a very positive frame of mind, knowing that something could be done and that she did not have to live with it. She came to see me some three weeks later. The swellings had disappeared, she was sleeping through the night and the pain was a thing of the past.

Some time later she was so busy with work, running a home, being a mother etc that she wandered from the straight and narrow and very quickly all the symptoms returned. She was told in no uncertain terms that she was, 'the boss' and if she wished to stay well the ball was very firmly in her court. I can diagnose, test, tell you all the pitfalls and put you on the right road to recovery but ultimately it rests with you. There is a saying I use with patients that I feel expresses it well – "Your body is the church in which you worship. How you worship is entirely up to you."

YOU DO NOT HAVE TO LIVE WITH ARTHRITIS!

Pesticides, Sprays

If you know anything about modern food production you will not need me to tell you that pesticides and sprays are in constant use. I referred earlier to the pesticides and sprays being used on pastureland, nitrites, nitrates, growth promoters, weed killers etc. The cattle feed on this and it ends up in our meat and milk. Weed killers are used to spray the potato crop while growing and again when they are put down for storage, and now of course GM Foods being used in cattle feed.

When my wife was asked, several years or so ago, and as a favour for a friend of ours, to collect the pesticides for his potato crop she had to sign three poison forms. A patient of mine is a very large potato grower in Kent, and when I mentioned about not eating the potato skins when baked, the reply I received was, "don't be silly, we would not eat those, we have a large patch for our own consumption".

Buy ORGANIC!! Your apples are sprayed so often it is unbelievable, and I have yet to test a patient who does not react to apple skin. Buy ORGANIC!! If they are not organic then please make sure you peel them. I am beginning to sound like a one-man advertising campaign for the Soil Association. They do an admirable job and you will see the Soil Association logo on foods that are acceptably organic. But that is not the reason I am mentioning these things, I am referring to clinical reactions, not just test results, but also the reports I receive from patients who have ingested something unsuitable. These reactions can be quite severe and often take as long as five days to clear the system and as long as three weeks for balanced health to return. So beware!! I would like to quote from a book called 'The Pesticide Conspiracy' by Professor Robert Van Den Bosch, it is the last page, *"Nature is emitting signals warning us that under the existing format the future is ominous. She is saying tha we cannot continue our attempts to ruthlessly dominate her and that if we persist disaster is in the offing. She has many voices, and of the clearest is that of the insects. The insects have already told us that we cannot overwhelm them and that there has been a price to pay in trying.*

But, Nature has other voices and, if we listen carefully, we can hear these additional warnings too: the voices of the trees in the crashing forests before an assault of axes, the later rumble of a mudslide as a cloudburst sweeps the denuded mountainside, the voice of the soil in the crunch of the alkali beneath the boots of a farmer pacing his land ruined by bad irrigation; the voice of the water as it roars crystal clear through the pen stocks of a mighty dam, leaving behind the nutrients that once nourished a great floodplain and fed a vast fishery; the voice of the wind as it hisses with a load of dust whipped from the topsoil of half a county.

Yes, the voices of Nature are quite easy to hear - if we will only listen. The question is, will we? And if we do, can we overcome our corrupt ways and marshal our efforts to collaborate with Nature as her brightest child and shepherd of Earth's life system? If not, it is almost certain that things will worsen for Nature, but even more so for us. Then at a certain point in time we may no longer be able to cope with the adversity and we will perish. But Nature will survive, and so, too, will the insects, her most successful children. And as a final bit of irony, it will be the insects that polish the bones of the very last of us to fall."

This was written and published in 1978. It does not take a lot of imagination to realise how prophetic these words were .Look at the threat we are under with the extinction of so many bee colonies. For thirty two years later we are seeing the natural resources of this world threatened, and the natural kingdom occupying the land and the sea being polluted to the point of extinction. Is it really surprising that fishermen patients of mine tell me that they would never touch the fish, or let their families do so, because they are so diseased through pollution. Potato growers who will not eat the produce they sell to the public, apple growers who save private orchards for their own consumption, the list is endless. Just consider the billions of pounds spent on additives and preservatives in this country alone, and you will see why there are cartels to protect them, and intentionally deprive you of the information that is rightly yours.(Conspiracy at its worst).

It really depends on you the public demanding NATURAL foods, uncontaminated by pesticides and sprays, additives and preservatives, genetically engineered, or irradiated so that those in power will listen and act upon the pressure you exert. Even politicians realise that it is the public that put them in office, so contact your local Member of Parliament if you have a complaint.

Drugs and Arthritis

N.S.A.I.D.s. Non Steroidal Anti - Inflammatory Drugs.

The first thing to notice is they are drugs. I have not come across one drug that does not have one or more side effects, or contra indications. Look in MIMS, Monthly Index of Medical Specialities. Have you noticed the portent of the title? Monthly Index- why on earth do we need a monthly index of drugs available for prescription by a GP? I have had it pointed out to me by a dear pharmacist friend of mine that I am nit picking, "as most journals update once a month". This may apply to drug bulletins but not to Nutritional Journals or alternative medications. I think you know as well as I do that new drugs, or old drugs under a new name, are introduced every month. Old drugs are taken *off* for one reason or another, such as Opren referred to earlier. What a blessing that it was removed before too much damage was done. As I was saying, look in MIMS and there is not one drug that does not have an addendum that states quite clearly 'side effects'. The most common side effect I have come across is that all NSAIDs cause disturbance to the digestive system, or even stomach ulceration. Prolonged use of these drugs can lead to haemorrhaging, you will often find that when these drugs are prescribed you will also be given Gaviscon or Zantac or another antacid to combat the symptoms, or even in combination with Misoprostol, Napratec or Arthrotec - listed under side effects with Misoprostol are gastro-intestinal upset and abdominal pain.

Another very important factor as far as I am concerned is that all NSAIDs, contain lactose. It is quite possible that if you ask your GP for an alternative many will prescribe the generic alternative Diclofenac Retard and these still can contain lactose. Always check the ingredients on the instruction leaflet contained in all drug packets these days. I take a monthly newsletter called "What Doctors Don't Tell You" (WDDTY). If any of you reading this book are interested in caring for your own, or your families health, I would strongly recommend you subscribe to this magazine. I will give the address in the 'Useful Addresses' section in the rear of this book. If you are only interested in the arthritic condition I strongly recommend you to send for the special pack which contains :- ARTHRITIS; THE PRICE OF PAINKILLERS and ARTHRITIS; SECOND LINE TERRORS.

Once you have read these you will see why I recommend that publication.

NSAIDs in particular mask the symptoms, reducing the pain level and some inflammation but allowing the condition to rage throughout the whole system unchecked. Think carefully about this. Is pain there for a reason? Of course it is. It is nature's way of telling you that something is wrong with the system, there is dis - ease. The drugs mask the pain and lull you into a false sense of security. Bear in mind that whilst drugs mask the pain the disease continues to advance and in time higher doses of the drugs are required. Whilst my treatment may not always be a total cure the symptoms do disappear and the condition does not worsen. In fact, in most cases it improves considerably.

I know the pain of arthritis and I also know how easy it is to take drugs to give you some rest from the pain and allow you to sleep. Do think very carefully before doing so and, if necessary, go to your library and look up the drug and its side effects. Bearing in mind that it only masks the symptoms. You, or any of your loved ones that are suffering and taking NSAIDs should check with your G. P. what the side effects are and if there could be long lasting damage? Remind yourselves and them:

YOU DO NOT HAVE TO LIVE WITH ARTHRITIS!!

Rheumatologists are beginning to routinely prescribe an alarming range of drugs whose side effects range from death, blindness, cancer and mental disorders. Many of these drugs are powerful immune-suppressants and cell blockers. Now, stop!! Take a deep breath and carefully read that last sentence again. Does anything strike you as odd? I am sure you have realised that the one thing that we need to fight infection of any kind is a healthy immune system and a healthy cell structure, yet here you are being prescribed drugs, by a rheumatologist who is a specialist in his field, that are the very things that are going to suppress that which you should be restoring and preserving. Can this possibly be the route to take? I certainly would not take it and I certainly would not advise one of my patients to follow it; as in my opinion it can only lead to disaster in the long term. I do grant however that in the short term it may offer some relief if the condition is extremely severe.

So many of these drugs now being prescribed for arthritis were never meant for this condition in the first place and are prescribed on a purely speculative basis. They might help. There are no mights, ifs, or buts in the course of the treatment I am recommending you to follow. It is not always easy, it is not always convenient, it certainly is not the soft option but it is a **SAFE** one. Let us look at some of these drugs: -

Methotrexate - Cytotoxic Drug

This drug in the wrong hands is a potential killer, causing liver and kidney damage, lung disease, gastro intestinal distress and bone marrow suppression.(Physicians Desk Reference, 1992, PDR, the US drugs reference bible), reports deaths among patients on the drug.

It stresses that the drug should only be given by "physicians whose knowledge and experience included the use of antimetabolite therapy."(Substances which fundamentally change the body's metabolism). As you can see it is a very powerful drug. When taken with other drugs such as NSAIDs they form a lethal cocktail. Methotrexate is one of a family of drugs called SAARDs, (slow acting anti-rheumatic drugs). These are considered as second line treatments. What exactly does that mean? It means that the first line treatments of choice have not worked effectively and something is needed to slow the condition down and hopefully prevent further damage to the joints.

Penicillamine

As the name suggests this is a component of penicillin and was developed originally to treat Wilson's disease (copper accumulation in the liver). For the arthritic condition the daily maintenance dose can be as high as 750mg, although the patient is usually started at 125mg and 250mg to test for adverse reactions. As usual there are side effects and the most common ones are: - skin rash, mouth ulcers, loss of taste and a more serious reaction can occur where there are skin eruptions. The treatment should be stopped immediately. The blood disorder thrombocytopenia is common and can be severe, *(Drugs and Therapeutic Bulletin,* 1993:3 1:18).

Sulfasalazine

Sulfasalazine is one of the family of drugs which block the growth of cells. Serious side effects include bone marrow suppression, increased risk of infection, infertility, nausea, vomiting, epigastric pain, headache, rashes, cancer and defects in the embryo. (G.W. Cannon & J.R. Ward, "Arthritis and Allied Conditions", Lea & Febiger, Philadelphia, 1989). The drug was originally developed to treat ulcerative colitis and Crohns disease. (ABPI Compendium Data Sheet, 1993-4).

Chloroquine/Hydroxychloroquine

These are anti-malaria drugs that, through trial and error, have been found to have some beneficial effects on rheumatoid arthritis. Common side effects include tinnitus, insomnia, hyperactivity and anaemia, gastro intestinal disturbance and headache.

Cyclosporin

This immunosuppressant, originally developed to stop the body from rejecting transplant organs, is the current flavour of the month in medicine. It is used to treat every disease doctors otherwise don't know how to handle. It acts by lowering the immune system T-Cells and should be used in treating rheumatoid arthritis only when the condition is life threatening.

Other immunosuppressants that may be recommended include Azathioprine and Cyclophosphamide, although they come with the same high risks. None are licensed in the United Kingdom for the treatment of arthritis, although they are being investigated.

Should we really be looking at suppressants of the immune system, particularly when they are only being investigated? I think not. We should be looking for the causatory 'trigger' of the breakdown of the immune system, and once determined, to eliminate it from the diet and allow the immune system to recover naturally, which thankfully it does, and more speedily with some help and support.

Steroids

After immunosuppressants, steroids are the most controversial - and possibly the most damaging treatments available for arthritis. Steroid overuse in the 1950's to treat arthritis and the horrors that came from it has put paid to the treatment among those Doctors with long memories. The Medical Research Council trial in 1960 concluded that the risks outweighed the benefits. The side effects of the glucocorticoids - which include cortisol, cortisone, prednisilone and dexamethasone - are many and various. These include the suppression of the immune system, osteoporosis, muscular dystrophy, peptic ulcer, psychiatric disorders, infections and eye problems (T.W.Behrens and J.S. Goodwin, *Arthritis and Allied Conditions,* Lea & Febiger, Philadelphia 1989).

I wish that I could agree with the above statement that most have learnt from the 1950s. I saw patients every week who were on steroids, mainly Prednisilone, and some have been on it for as long as five years. One only has to look at these patients and see the damage that has been done to realise how suppressing the immune system fools the body and masks the pain while destroying kidney and liver function and causing deterioration of the bone structure, osteoporosis!!.

However, I have to be honest and say that my impression is that rheumatologists are becoming less eager to put patients on steroids long term these days. Let us hope that trend continues and, perhaps one can hope that one bright day, they may start looking for the cause, instead of looking for a drug to suppress it. It will not happen in my days in practice as those days are already gone, but hopefully this century. **YOU DO NOT HAVE TO LIVE WITH ARTHRITIS!!!**

Dear Mr Davies,

Just to say "thank you" seems so inadequate an expression for giving me back my health.

At 55 I had written myself off as a normal healthy person, finished with an active life and had put my business on the market for sale and now, only six weeks after our consultation, I am going to expand the business and have bought a motor caravan and am going on a long tour of Scotland early next year

To be able to rise early in the morning, full of good health, and look forward to the challenge of each new day is to know that good health is life's greatest gift.

I can never thank you enough for giving back to me that great gift of good health but, be assured, you have my eternal gratitude

Mr P.C.
Newbury
Berkshire

This man expanded his businesses three fold.

Antibiotics

When penicillin was discovered it was thought we had a magic bullet. It would kill all bacteria and cure all bacterial infections. Life would be so wonderful if it was as simple as that. Pop a pill and all will be well. Of course it did not work like that and unfortunately we have had the hard lesson to learn, that by using antibiotics as the cure-all, the bullet has turned on us and shot us in the foot. Bacteria learn to adapt and become resistant, our former wonder drugs are now all but useless. Did you realise that antibiotics only treat bacteria. Many of the deadly infections today are caused by viruses and antibiotics are useless against them. We can be infected by fungi too, and antibiotics encourage fungal growth. Consider this point carefully please: - Every time you take an antibiotic you are giving the bacteria around you a new opportunity to develop resistance. Remember my comments about organic food - every time you eat milk, cheese, eggs and most meats, unless they are organic, you are being exposed to antibiotics. Livestock are given daily doses virtually from birth, because antibiotics are growth promoters, and keep milk and eggs fresh for much longer, thus increasing farmer's profits.

So, what is the consequence? Fewer and fewer antibiotics are effective against deadly infections. Patients who contract serious infections like pneumonia, or pick up a hospital infection like the deadly staphylococcus, often die because the bacteria are so resistant. The recent E-Coli outbreak in Scotland is a typical example. In America, New York in particular, tuberculosis is becoming epidemic, it is quoted as affecting as many as 1 in 3 of the population, and it is antibiotic resistant. Do not be complacent it is also making a comeback in the United Kingdom too.

Because of antibiotic abuse we have lost the 'war'. Remember the last major outbreak of Influenza in this country. It was in the winter of 1996/7 and thousands of people were affected. It lingered on for months and what were many told when they went to their GP? "Well, you have influenza but there is nothing I can do for you or give you as they do not work, so go home and it will burn itself out eventually". I do not wish to sound anti GP because if there were to be a secondary infection, or a suspicion of it, then antibiotics would be prescribed. But it really does not inspire confidence when it is publicly stated that antibiotics are not effective in these viral conditions. Think long and hard please, there are alternative ways of approaching illness of any kind; protecting and strengthening the immune system is one way of doing just that. What happens when we get a scare that chicken flu (never happened) or swine flu (never happened), we are told there are vaccines available, and what are the ingredients of these vaccines? Who makes the money? The pharmaceutical companies in every single case. If they are not used in this country as with Tamiflu then they are shipped to countries such as Africa.

Alexander Fleming, who discovered penicillin warned nearly a century ago that overuse of antibiotics would create resistant bacteria.

Alternatives

Yes, there are some very good ones. I can remember recently attending a meeting where the general body of the public were against a road being driven across the only piece of Green Wedge left in Taunton and a local planning officer stood up and said, "I am sure you are right, the Green Wedge should be preserved, but do not criticise the existing plans unless you have an alternative". Well, I have certainly criticised the use of drugs for many years and thankfully I can suggest alternatives. They are certainly many and varied and I have tried most of them over the years, on myself and my patients, with varying degrees of success. However in the last three years the most effective, and therefore the most successful, are the first two mentioned. These are not drugs but natural supplements.

Glucosamine Sulphate

Tissues in and around the joints get damaged because the lubricating synovial fluids in the joint spaces become thin and watery instead of being thick and elastic. There is a loss of the natural cushioning and consequently the bones and the lining cartilages collide and scrape together inside the joint space. A loss of cushioning by watery bursae allows tendons to rub against the hard edges of the bones. Cartilage starts to erode and problems arise.

Glucosamine sulphate helps to restore the thick, gelatinous nature of the fluids and tissues in and around the joints and in between the vertebrae. N-Acetyl Glucosamine and Glucosamine Sulphate are among the types of biological chemicals that form hyaluronic acid, a major cushioning ingredient of the joint fluids and surrounding tissues.

Glucosamine sulphate may therefore give good results, in a short period of time, for the following indications: -

- degeneration, swelling and inflammation of the synovial fluids.
- osteo-arthritis during recovery of injuries, after operations and during recuperation.
- damage to and inflammation of the attachment muscles.
- dystrophy of joints associated with ageing.
- injury and loss of elasticity of intervertebral discs.
- use preventively in cases of overburdening of the joints for example, intensive sport, poor work posture, heavy lifting, generally in ageing and so on.

I have used this product for several years now and the results in the main have been most encouraging. There has been the odd patient who reported that it appeared to upset the stomach so it was discontinued. There is a very good reason for this as I shall explain later. If you try any alternative supplements and they appear to cause a reaction then discontinue immediately and have a word with your practitioner. This the last three product is available from: - Hildreth & Cocker 0800 316 6714, or The Nutri Centre. 0207 436 5122.

B-Alive

This product has revolutionised the recovery of my patients for years, surpassing anything I had used previously. I take two tablets daily every day and will continue to do so ad infinitum. I recommend all my lady patients over the age of thirty five to take it to prevent osteoporosis, rather than HRT the so called elixir of life for women in the menopause, more of which in a moment. There is an excellent booklet called "Away With Arthritis" written by the man who helped to formulate the product, Dr Rex Newnham. You will find his name and address in the useful addresses section at the rear of this book. It is an excellent read and explains how the condition occurs, what B-Alive does to ameliorate the condition and how it does it. The firm that supplies B-Alive in this country, and the booklet, are Hildreth & Cocker, 0800 316 6714.

B-Alive is sold under different names in various countries. In the United States it is known as Osteo Trace and is available as follows: - in OHIO and the surrounds from Dr Don Brenn, 1535 N-Limestone St, Springfield, OH 45503. Tel: 513 3903557.

CALIFORNIA - Mumme Enterprises, 1321, Meridian Aye, South Pasadena, CA 91030. Tel: 213 2554550.

NEW ZEALAND - BORE-REX is on sale at most health shops throughout the country and BOREXON is available from many chemists. If you have any problems obtaining these products then try the wholesalers, Bore-Rex New Zealand, P0 58-728, Greenmount, Auckland. Tel: 09 274 1630.

SOUTH AFRICA - RAY-REX tablets are available at most good pharmacies, failing that from: Jacobs Pharmacy, P0 Box 2562, Durban, 4000.

Initially these boron supplements were sold under the name Bore-Rex, but that name was too close to other registered trademarks in some other countries, so the name had to be changed. However, these are the only boron supplement tablets that have been submitted to and passed hospital trial. They were shown to be effective with 70% of cases that completed the trial and these were all severe cases with the average age of 64. When younger people use these products as a preventive measure we can expect nearly 100% effectiveness.

Quite rightly Rex states in his booklet, 'that if people were encouraged to prevent their illness in the first place there would be no need for hospitals. Healthy people do not need hospitals".

Quite naturally I would agree with him. This entire book is really all about the prevention of, or recovery from, arthritis without the need to use drugs. I must say though, as it is with many supplements, it is 'horses for courses'. Some need as many as six daily to start then reduce down to two to three daily, whereas some patients can only cope with one daily. Thank goodness we are all different. If you do have an adverse reaction, do not give up completely, leave them alone for five days, then introduce half a tablet daily for a week, then increase at a half tablet each time until you reach the recommended dosage. You should find that it works effectively.

Flax Oil

I have recommended this to patients for a long time, particularly organic flax or hemp oil. You will also find that throughout this book I will relax into the modern idiom and abbreviate it wherever possible to FO .Why is it necessary to be so pedantic as to say two hours after the evening meal? For a very good reason. We try to cheat the liver! Because the liver is the 'sponge' or the 'pantry' of the body. As arthritics we need to cheat the liver and create a diversion by eating our evening meal. The liver is then busy digesting and disseminating to other organs. While it is busy doing this, two hours after the evening meal, we take the FO and sneak it past the liver so that it can help to build new tissues throughout the body. In so doing it delivers oil to the joint linings and cartilage to check osteo and rheumatoid arthritis. It can fill the sac with oil in bursitis, lubricate the muscles in myolitis, cover the nerves with oil in neuritis and nourish the connective tissue in fibrositis. Hemp oil is also very beneficial and is in 2010 the practitioners oil of choice.

Evening Primrose Oil

A report in the Lancet reveals that evening primrose oil is effective for a substantial number of patients suffering from rheumatoid arthritis and is therefore worth considering as a nutritional supplement.

There are various brands on the market and you must check to ensure that it states on the ingredients, pure evening primrose oil, no padders, fillers etc; the one that has been most effective for me is called GLA - Gamma Linolenic Acid from Biocare Ltd. 0121 433 3727. One, or at the most two of these, daily is usually enough to relieve the symptoms.

In recommending these products I do not wish to imply that other products on the market are not suitable. There are many, and I have tried most of them, but I have found the products I mention to be the ones that have produced the best results for me.

I mentioned earlier The Nutri Centre,7, Park Crescent, London. WiN 3HE. This centre stocks most of the leading brands of supplements available today and I am sure a phone call to discuss the matter would be met with a helpful response and good advice.0207 436 5122.

Whilst on the subject of supplements, it has become increasingly evident over the last few years that there is a definite link between arthritis and candidiasis - Candida Albicans. In simplistic terms this means an over population of candida albicans in the gut and causing a dysbiosis, an imbalance. Certainly the parasite most commonly associated with arthritis is Endolimax Nana. If treated correctly relief can be obtained quite quickly, the most badly affected are young children. The most recent estimate is 28 million cases in America.

While on the subject of the relationship between arthritis and candida it is important to state the current findings. Once the arthritic diet, with the elimination of allergens, has been carried out for three weeks and there is no sign of any improvement then obviously one starts to look for possible culprits. As it is recommended on the arthritis diet to take molasses, a pure sugar derivative, and the fruit is limitless, then, as a precaution the molasses is eliminated, along with honey, mushrooms and root vegetables, and the fruit limited to apple, pear and banana for a further three weeks to see if the condition responds. If it does not respond then you must contact your practitioner. They will carry out tests to see if there is a pre-disposing candidiasis and advise you which medication to take. I would certainly ask for a fecal sample, send it off to the laboratory, and ascertain if the parasite Endolimax Nana or candida were evident. If the results are positive and medication is prescribed it is amazing how quickly the condition responds.

So, if you have arthritis, have tried the diet for at least six weeks and nothing has happened to improve the condition, do not give up. There is always a reason. Find a practitioner near to you, explain what you have done, and give them a chance to correct things, you should improve within weeks.

I referred earlier to the product B-Alive that has helped so many of my patients over the last twenty years and to the man responsible for this product, Rex. E. Newnham Ph.D. DO. N.D. There is an explanatory leaflet that Hildreth & Cocker send out with B-Alive so those of you that order it will be familiarised with the product. However I think it will do no harm to put some of that leaflet information into this book, at least you will have a good flavour of what the product does.

Nutrients For Relieving Arthritis

BORON is essential for all green plants and when the content of boron in the plant gets down to about 1 part per million those plants fail to grow properly; apples become brown and fibrous or corky, potatoes develop hollows with brown edges, brassicas develop hollow stems and poorly formed buds. Until the 1960s no one had been able to show any need for boron in man or animal, but then it was discovered that boron would correct much arthritis, both rheumatoid arthritis (RA) and osteoarthritis (OA). The first paper announcing this was in 1979 (Newnham R.E., *Boron Beats Arthritis,* ANZAAS, Australian Academy of Science, Canberra, 1979).

Dr Forrest Nielsen, of the US Human Research Centre in North Dakota, in 1987 tried boron on post-menopausal women. These women, on a typical institutionalised diet that contained only 0.25mg boron a day, were losing calcium at the rate of 117mg a day. When they were given a boron supplement of 3mg the calcium loss dropped to 64mg a day (Nielsen FH, Hunt CD, Mullen LM, Hunt JR: *Effect of Dietary Boron on Mineral, Estrogen and Testosterone Metabolism in Post-Menopausal Women,* N. Dakota Acad. of Sc., 1987).

A pilot clinical trial was started in Melbourne in 1983 and after 5 years it was completed. It was designed for OA patients only and of those that completed the trial 70% responded favourably when using boron but only 12% on placebo (Prayers RL, Rennie GC, Newnham RE, *Boron and Arthritis: The Results of a Double Blind Pilot Study,* J of Nutritional Medicine,1.1990). In this trial some people apparently also had RA and they opted out of the trial.

RA patients invariably suffer an early aggravation or Herxheimer reaction after the first week or two, but then after another two or three weeks they normally get quite better. Even people whose fingers and hands were bent and twisted so as to be really useless were able to sew and knit or weave after treatment with boron. Systemic lupus erythematosus is a severe form of RA and this responds just as well. Young children with Still's disease or juvenile arthritis will get quite better in just a few days.

OA patients will recover without any aggravation. OA often comes after severe damage to joints, such as found in footballers and those who drive earth moving machinery. Some respond in just a few days but generally speaking those under 60 respond in the first month, those in their 60s take 2 months, those in their 70s take 3 months and those in their 80s and 90s can take over 3 months.

We know that fluoride will give dental fluorosis when there is an unevenness in the enamel of the teeth but this also occurs in every bone of the body as skeletal fluorosis. People in some parts of India and Africa who have too much natural fluoride have endemic fluorosis and can hardly stand up or work. Boron is the natural antagonist to fluoride. People who drink fluoridated water will develop skeletal fluorosis, but their doctors were never taught about this and they just call it arthritis. This is corrected with boron.

Those with broken bones are advised to take a boron supplement as boron works through the parathyroid to speed up bone mineralisation. Broken bones will heal in half the normal time when boron is taken quickly after the accident. A sheep dog was run over and sustained a broken pelvis, he was not really expected to live, but he was put on boron and is now back at work, just as lively as ever. Horses have also recovered from fractures.

When a person has arthritis it is wise to take 9mg a day and then reduce it to 3mg a day a month after all arthritic symptoms have gone. This is the maintenance dose to prevent recurrence of the trouble. Those with Osteoporosis are advised to take 3mg a day, after first using 3 tablets a day for 3 months.

It is wise to only use boron in a form that has been tested and proven in a proper hospital trial. Some tablets, for example, contain chelated boron and this means that the boron is tightly attached to some other organic molecule. We want the boron readily available and not tightly combined to anything. Nielsen's work in the USA has shown that boron will naturally raise the level of hormones in the body to the normal level. (Hormone replacement therapy or HRT is used by some people to try to overcome the effects of osteoporosis, but there is risk of cancer with the therapy).

Boron is not stored in the body so frequent small doses are required, this being more efficacious than one larger dose. Soil that has had much chemical fertiliser tends to have less available boron so that the plant foods grown on these soils are less nutritious. A good apple grown without chemicals can have 10mg of boron but the average commercial apple often has less than 1mg of boron. It is our food production system that affects uptake of trace minerals and is responsible for more arthritis than 100 years ago.

Analysis has shown that bones and teeth from patients with RA contain less boron than is found in healthy people (Ward, NI "The Determination of Boron in Biological Materials by Neutron Radiation and Prompt Gamma-Ray Spectrometry". Journal of Radio-analytical and Nuclear Chemistry, 110.2, 1987).

ESSENTIAL VITAMINS AND MINERALS

Magnesite is a natural magnesium mineral which is essential for good bone structure. It is essential for the metabolism of vitamin B6 and enters into many enzyme processes in the body. The parathyroids require magnesium for the proper control of calcium in the bones. (See Shils ME. 1976 Magnesium Deficiency and Calcium and Parathyroid Interrelations P.23-46 in Trace Elements in Health and Disease Vol. 2 Prasad and Oberleas Academic Press NY).

Pyridoxine/Vitamin B6 has been used to treat rheumatism as it reduces edema, joint stiffness, pain and sensory numbness, especially in the arms. (Dr. Ellis, *The Doctor's Report* 1973).

Zinc is essential for many bodily functions, especially for the proper cross linking of connective tissue in cartilage, and for its regeneration (See Prasad and Oberleas as above).

Silica or Diatomite contains silicon which is essential for normal growth in all animals and man. Its deficiency causes depressed growth and abnormal bone formation. It is essential for mucopolysaccharide metabolism and proper cartilage formation (See Davis N.T. 1981. *An Appraisal of the Newer Trace Elements* P. 173-174 in *Trace Element Deficiency; Metabolic and Physiological Consequences.* Ed. Fowden, Garton and Mills. Royal Soc. London).

Vitamin B3 Niacin is a component of 2 co-enzymes, NAD and NADP, essential for cell respiration as well as being involved in fat and protein synthesis and is reported to help arthritic conditions. (Doctor Hoffer, *The Complete Book of Vitamins,* 1977).

Pantothenate - **Vitamin B5** has been used to treat rheumatism as it aids tissue repair. Rheumatoid arthritics have low blood levels of this vitamin according to Drs Barton- Wright and Elliot (*Lancet,* October 1963).

Kelp is rich in iodine and boron; both these help to stimulate the parathyroid glands which in turn control the calcium in bones.

Devil's Claw is an African herb that has long been recognised as useful for arthritis.

Manganese is essential for many enzyme processes and in proper use of many of the B Vitamins, which in turn help arthritic conditions. Muscular rheumatism is helped by manganese. Zinc and manganese work together to control the body levels of other heavy metals. It is found mainly in whole grains and green leaf vegetables.

Copper is essential for the proper formation of haemoglobin and red blood cells. Arthritics need adequate blood to carry around the necessary minerals and other bone forming substances. Cartilage must also be repaired and blood helps here. Some elderly people tend towards anaemia so the blood must be built up in order to help them properly. Very little is needed but that small amount is necessary.

Calcium Fluoride is very sparingly soluble but it is absorbed through the intestine. When 117 incorporated into the bones as calcium fluoroapatite it gives hardness and strength to the bone crystals. It stimulates osteoblastic activity and so helps in formation of new bone, especially after damage. Very little is needed but it certainly helps in many cases of osteoarthritis, rheumatoid arthritis, osteoporosis and ankylosing spondylitis. (See Blackmores Prescribers Reference A.8.1).

Molybdenum helps to prevent dental caries which are really poor bone growth of the teeth, so other bones are likely to be similarly affected. Together with zinc it helps to counter the effect of other heavy metals. It is found in whole grains, seeds, beans, nuts and eggs.

Selenium is an anti-oxidant and will aid in the metabolism of Vitamin E. It is essential for the proper functioning of muscles and is a must for muscular rheumatism. It is present in garlic, whole grains, meat and eggs. Men and animals cannot live without it but we only need 200 micro grams daily. Remember many arthritics cannot break down wholemeal flour.

Cobalt is part of the Vitamin B12 or hydroxycobalamin. We need very little of it but it is essential for the liver and proper blood formation. It is present in meat foods, especially liver (organic only) and vegetarians are often short of this vitamin. Its presence ensures better growth and resistance to disease.

Pregnancy makes big demands on the body's reserves of this vitamin because the developing foetus must get it for proper growth.

Bee Pollen is a natural source of boron and is rich in trace elements.

Equisetum/Horse Tail is a herb rich in silica and this helps to harden bones.

Cod Liver Oil and Hemp oil are rich in Vitamin D which is essential for good bone formation, growth and maintenance. Young people often get sufficient by exposure to sunshine, but the elderly and those living in northern climes can need a supplement. Oily fish such as herring, cod and mackerel have this vitamin in the proper natural form that does not adversely affect anyone.

Linseed Oil/Flax Oil is also a rich source of Omega 3 EFA and would be beneficial taken in conjunction with **a** reduced dosage of cod liver oil.

A NUTRITIONAL SUPPLEMENTARY APPROACH TO THE RESTORATION OF DEGENERATED CONNECTIVE JOINT TISSUES IN OSTEOARTHRITIS AND RHEUMATOID ARTHRITIS by Brian Hildreth T.T.C, C.H.R., C.H..F.

"***Osteoarthritis*** *is a degenerative disease and is associated with getting older. It's the 'wear and tear' arthritis that is usually characterised by the degeneration of joint cartilage. . . .As the cartilage and the other tissues around the joint break down the joint becomes less comfortable and more difficult to move...*"

"***Rheumatoid arthritis*** *is the most crippling of all the arthritis conditions and appears to do most of its damage to the joints. Unfortunately it also damages the body's connective tissues that support the bones and internal organs. ..*" (Robert C Atkins M.D. *How to Treat Your Medical Condition Without Drugs* 1981).

In both forms of arthritis, as simply and concisely stated in the quotations above, it is the breakdown and degeneration of the connective tissues in the joints (synovial membrane, hyaline cartilage, fibro-cartilage) without their replacement, which leads to its crippling effects. The degeneration is particularly painful and crippling when it is the fibro -cartilage which forms the vertebral discs between the bones of the spinal vertebrae which is involved.

Osteoarthritis is a degenerative non-flammatory disease which principally affects the synovial (freely movable) joints.

As the disease progresses the articular cartilage gradually becomes thinner as its removal becomes faster than its replacement rate. As a result of this cartilaginous thinning the articular surface of the bones come in contact and consequent bone degeneration is the inevitable outcome.

Rheumatoid arthritis is an inflammatory disease which produces a variety of secondary changes in the body together with erosion of the articular cartilage of the synovial joints. There has been for some time controversy regarding the possibility of reversing this change in the cartilage and connective tissues through dietary measures. This argument also extends to the treatment of osteoarthritis. **However there is now a considerable body of evidence showing that, provided rigid dietary constraints are followed together with appropriate mineral and vitamin supplements, it is possible to rebuild degenerative tissues provided the treatment is maintained over a considerable time span.**

The Dietary Problem

For a dietary approach to the treatment of both forms of arthritis to be successful it must obviously supply the correct nutrients needed for connective tissue rebuilding and these nutrients must be of such a composition that the body utilises them specifically for their intended purpose.

In the past this 'specificity' of nutritional requirements has proved to be a difficult factor in devising anti-arthritis diets and many are characterised by stringent lists of foods to avoid together with dietary regimes often of a restrictive nature. The dietary regimen recommended in this book are tailored to those patients who have been tested and the diet adjusted accordingly, I do not consider them to be stringent providing they obtain their objective, freedom of pain and recuperation of bones and tissue rebuilding.

Allergic reactions to various foodstuffs are a factor which **must** be taken into account and obviated from any diet but, once all considerations have been observed, it is the actual dietary intake which must be able to supply the correct nutrients if it is to be efficacious from a therapeutic point of view. This is the dietary problem. Eliminating particular foodstuffs is not difficult but replacing them with dietary elements which will achieve the **best results possible is not easy, and this is why it is recommended you see a Clinical Ecologist.** Preferably one trained by me.

At the heart of the problem is the major nutritional question - what must an arthritic sufferer have in his or her diet which will supply exactly the right nutrients for restoration of degenerated, and degenerating, connective tissue? There now appears to be no doubt that there is a group of essential nutrients for arthritic disease.

The nutrients required are a combination of amino-sugar-containing polysaccharides known as mucopolysaccharides / glycosaminoglycans (GAGs). (Glucosamine.)

Connective Tissue Composition

Until recently connective tissue and its structure has not received a great deal of attention. Fortunately this situation has changed and now a considerable amount of research has been devoted to it.

Its chemical structure is far more complex than originally thought and it has been found to consist of mucopolycsaccharides (GAGs), hyaluronic acid, chondroitin sulphuric acid, chondroitin sulphate, chondroitin, and various proteins containing large amounts of the amino acid tyrosine.

One of these constituents of connective tissue with an important relationship to chondroitin sulphate is collagen, the basic material of fibrous tissue which forms the ligaments which bind bones together, which forms the outer protective covering of the bone (periosteum), protects some organs such as the kidneys and the lymph nodes and forms muscle sheaths (fascia) which extend beyond the muscle to form the tendon which attaches muscle to bone.

The structure and composition of the connective tissue is functionally related to the circulatory system and the efficiency of the circulation determines the transport of materials to it and the drainage of materials from it.

Among these materials (oestrogen, androgens, thyroxine, adrenoglucocorticoids, adrenomineralcorticoids) carried in the blood to permeate through the connective tissue is the all important chondroitin sulphate which builds up depleted connective tissue such as cartilage and synovial membranes. At the same time further important actions appear to be initiated with the inhibition of enzymatic breakdown of the collagen together with an enhancement fibrin dissolving enzymes. glucosamine/chondroitin sulphate thus appears to be a necessary constituent of any effective dietary programme applied to the treatment of osteoarthritis and rheumatoid arthritis, and this has been borne out in practice.

Taken at a daily rate of lOg of (20% glucosamine) powder 6-8 (95% glucosamine) capsules per day together with a suitable diet, arthritic sufferers with a long history of the disease (one female with acute symptoms for ten years) all showed dramatic improvement within three weeks of commencing the supplementation of their diet. As an added 'side effect' they all reported an increase in energy, but the main expression of improvement was increased freedom of joint movement with better mobility that included those with spinal problems

In a minority of patients there was reported increase in 'normal' joint pain for a period of approximately 48 hours after commencing use of the supplement. It appears that this is due to regenerative processes occurring and increased activity in the target area. It is emphasised that this is a temporary increase in discomfort and does not occur in all sufferers.

Clinical trials conducted to date show that chondroitin sulphate has a definite therapeutic action and any arthritis sufferer can only benefit from its application to their diet."

As with all scientific explanations it is possible to be baffled by technical jargon, and at times it is impossible to simplify it enough for same, however, I hope it has helped you to understand the process a little more than previously. Certainly the most important factor of all in my experience is to determine the causatory 'trigger' and the subsequent production of bradikinin. In simple terminology find the allergen, eliminate it and immediately the body will start to heal itself. However, the damage that has been done must be repaired - degeneration must be turned into regeneration and this where the use of B-Alive, glucosamine and chondroitin sulphate have proved so invaluable to me in my practice and the successful recovery of my patients.

I would like to finish this chapter on another case history, and some further information regarding Endolimax Nana. The case history first.

MR. A.F. from TORQUAY

This man presented with arthritis and asthma and is now perfectly well and working-in what I call a hazardous profession, dry cleaning and laundering. He first noticed the pain and swelling in 1991 and put up with it for six months before visiting his GP. He was informed it was arthritis and could be given pain killers but did not accept this. In February 1994 he consulted me and as well as the breathing problems he had pain and swelling in the knees, elbows, fingers and in his own words, "was particularly painful and could not walk up stairs without supporting myself, and I could not hold golf clubs!!" Being a fellow golfer, I know how frustrating that must have been. Within four weeks he was free of pain, the swelling had diminished and he has progressed favourably ever since. Inhalers are a thing of the past and he is fit and well. Again in his own words **"completely free of pain and tenderness"**,

YOU DO NOT HAVE TO LIVE WITH ARTHRITIS!!

Now for the information on this parasite **Endolimax Nana.** It is known to be the major parasite which produces reactive arthritis and, in my experience, it is only treatable by placing the patient on a candida diet along with the arthritic diet and treating the gut dysbiosis brought about by this parasite. The supplementation I have used to the greatest effect is as follows: Keep to the candida/arthritic diet and take HEP 194 to detox the liver, the poor old liver has to take the brunt of the detoxification process, and this is usually a tough time and in some cases the pain gets worse before it gets better. It is essential to measure the joint inflammation at this time so that an assessment can be made in three weeks. If all has gone reasonably well then commence the herbal parasite programme (HPP) listed in the chapter on Candidiasis. During this time a supplementation of Lactobaccilus bulgaricus (powder) should be taken at half teaspoon daily to replace the lost healthy bacteria. It is then absolutely essential to carry out the maintenance programme weekly, once you are free of pain and swelling apart from the maintenance day introduce B-Alive and Reflex.

Obviously as I have stated before every patient is different, but on average a period of two to three weeks on this regimen is sufficient to bring the condition under control. It is then essential to seal the gut and prevent any further incursion in to the bloodstream (Leaky Gut Syndrome). Enteroguard, for 10 days to 14 days as directed on tub.

Vegedophilus, to be continued one before breakfast for at least a further month. By this time the condition should be much improved and you should be able to go back on to the arthritic diet with no problems. The above supplementation is available from Biocare or the Nutri Centre previously mentioned.

I am a Psoritic arthritic. What this means is that I suffer from psoriasis, a skin condition which in many ways resembles ringworm, and affects all parts of the body. I have had it in my ears and eyes, and pustular arthritis on the feet, and jolly painful it is too. Do not be complacent about this condition either. It is a well-known and accepted fact within the medical fraternity that psoriasis and arthritis are bedfellows. One can lead to the other. So, if you have psoriasis take precautionary measures now, do not wait until arthritis strikes. Eliminate the dairy products first. If that does not work try the arthritic diet and, if that does not work, try the candida procedure. It will be worth it I assure you.

YOU DO NOT HAVE TO LIVE WITH ARTHRITIS!!

Chapter 16

Diet For Life

The title speaks for itself really. It is for life once you have discovered your basic allergens. I would much prefer to call it a way of eating. There are so many occasions where patients have kept strictly to the recommended guidelines, observed the benefits with recovery to full health and freedom from pain. So, human nature being what it is we now think that as we are well we can go off the rails a bit, it will not hurt!! Once you believe or assume that - you are in real trouble and heading for a big let-down, the reaction is almost instantaneous. The temptation is always there, when the first reaction is negative, to continue in that vein, this is the first step down the slippery slope. Please do not take that course. Let me try and explain the situation and why the reactions occur so quickly. As you detoxify and clear the system the adrenal glands, sitting on top of the kidneys like two healthy walnuts, respond, and behave as they should by producing adrenaline, cortisone, and histamine (ACH) to protect you and keep you on an even keel. When a suspect food is ingested the natural defences of the body leap into action and are able to cope. But if this is repeated too often the adrenal glands atrophy (shrink) and the toxins are released into the system again. So, please do not be fooled. Remember what I said about the three stages of the General Adaptation Syndrome? I would like to explain a typical reaction of the above scenario. Richard is a large well built man and if anything was carrying a little too much weight. He is a member of my golf club, and while playing in a match together, he mentioned that he was considering giving up golf because it was becoming too painful. I then asked him why this should be and he told me he had been diagnosed as having arthritis. The hands were so painful it was difficult to hold the clubs, and hurt every time he hit the ball.

I told him he did not have to give up golf, but if he was willing to give up certain foods and keep rigidly to a strict diet then he was to come and see me; this he duly did and we discovered his basic allergens and put him on the special diet. In a very short space of time the pain and swelling had disappeared, he had lost weight and felt much better.

This went on for some months until he informed me one day that the pain was back in his hands. I asked him if he had changed his diet in any way and he assured me he had not. I then asked if he had introduced anything new into his normal diet, only honey and sheep's yoghurt. Could the sheep's yoghurt be too rich for the liver to cope with? "More likely to be the honey as we as arthritics do not cope with sugar too well I told him." "I will cut them out and see what happens", he said. Three weeks later I saw Richard at the golf club and enquired how things were going, the reply was most encouraging, "fantastic thank you," he said. Needless to say I was much relieved but curious, so I asked "was it the honey?"- "well, not exactly he said," as you probably know I am a builder and I take two flasks of tea to work every day and I was putting six spoonfuls of sugar in each flask!!" An overload on the pancreas, initial reaction nil, adaptation for a week or two, then, Stage Three!! The immune system could not cope and back came the condition with a vengeance. Such a simple slip, but look at the disastrous results.

It is worth mentioning here that an alternative to milk such as Soya often contain a lot of sugar, DO CHECK THE INGREDIENTS. It really is never worth taking risks unless you are sure it is safe. If things begin to go wrong, no matter how simple it may seem, think carefully about a food or substance you may have recently introduced. I know by bitter experience that, once you are free of arthritic pain, there really is no urgency to return to that again. It is a terrifying thought.

So, on we go to the diet, and as I have said before I would much prefer to call it a way of eating. It appears to me that once you start altering a patient's food intake they are on a diet, so we shall call it that. Once you have established your basic allergens then it is a matter of keeping to the regimen for at least six weeks to see whether pain and swelling diminish. If all is well, then you know that this is the way forward and apart from the occasional treat, it is for life. I will come to occasional treats later, they are always better for the waiting aren't they?

I would like to include at this point a paragraph by the great Naturopath Harry Benjamin M.D. "By the very nature of the case, such quick and definite results as those which follow the treatment for simple rheumatism, cannot be expected, natural treatment holds out the only cure - or even partial cure that exists for them in the world today. Orthodox medical treatment, by means of injection or otherwise, is worse than useless where real cure is concerned. The sufferer from arthritis, more so than any other, can afford to no longer tamper with their diet if a cure - or even partial cure - is wished for."

When you realise that this statement was made in one of his books, more than fifty years ago, it makes you aware not only how profound that statement was. Just how much money has been wasted on arthritic research, which could have been spent more wisely researching the effect of food on the human system. The drug companies which fund these research projects would not like that. It would mean that anyone who had any respect for their body would not take drugs for fear of the known side effects, then where would the drug companies be? In recent years there has been more advice to cut back on red meat, watch fats and eat more vegetables, but it is not well publicised so most people remain unaware.

Listen to many general practitioners, certainly the majority of rheumatologists, and they will tell you quite categorically that food has nothing to do with arthritis at all. Yet if you ask at your

Pharmacy you will be given a leaflet called *A Patients Guide to Common Arthritic Conditions,* in it dietary advice is given. When you challenge GPs and Rheumatologists and ask them what research has been carried out they have no answer because, quite simply, no tests have ever been carried out in depth or superficially. It is dismissed out of hand. In all his years of study a doctor is provided with approximately six hours training on nutrition and diet and that only in recent years. Please do not think I am knocking doctors, in general, they do a splendid job under the incredible circumstances in which they work. I believe I am right in saying that a doctor is allowed within the confines of the National Health Service only 3-5 minutes per patient in the cities, marginally more in rural areas, for most consultations. This is to listen to what the patient is saying, test and diagnose, write a prescription or letter of referral, tab it into the computer - next patient please!! How can this possibly be sufficient time to diagnose or treat a condition as serious as arthritis? On the 23-3-2003, I listened to Professor Jonathan Brostoff saying how sad it was that, because doctors do not have enough nutritional and food allergy training, we are dealing with a National Ill Health Service whereas it could be so different. Professor Brostoff is an eminent Immunologist in London and is Patron of Action Against Allergy.

There are rules and guidelines to follow and, if you join a club and I hope you will join those of us that are now free of the dreadful symptoms of arthritis, what do you do? You abide by the rules, or you do not bother to join. So here we go - gird up your loins - be ready for a change of eating and remember please, raw and organic is best, lightly cooked and fresh is next best, frozen is third best and last of all tinned. Although having said that I have advised patients for years to eat fish and oily fish in particular and in most cases this has been no problem.

I am going to remind you again that the first seven to ten days of withdrawal are the worst. The most common complaint in the first twenty-four hours is a very nasty headache. Also remember we are all different so our recovery times are not going to be the same. So bear this in mind please and do not get disheartened if you are not free of pain in the first few weeks, give it at least six weeks and then, if nothing has changed, consult your naturopath, homeopath or nutritionist, (Clinical Ecologist).

The following is a list of your ENEMIES and POISONS:

Prepared foods and processed foods, Packaged deserts, Tinned soups, Tinned fruits, Tinned meats, Tinned vegetables, Tinned poultry, Cake, Sweets, Ice cream, Smoked fish and meats, salami, corned beef ,Packaged cereals, Bakery products, Spaghetti, Pasta, Refined rice, Noodles, Pizza, Coffee, Soft drinks, Jams, Jellies, Sugar and artificial sweeteners, Imitation dairy products, Fabricated foods, imitated, altered or semi-prepared by man, Wine, Beer, Liquor.

I know what you are going to say — "what is there left to eat?" The answer of course is a lot, Fresh fruit. Garden fresh vegetables, Delicious fish and selected meats, Natural cheeses, eggs, nuts and natural sweeteners, such as Xylitol.

Which would be your choice?

Apple pie and cream topped with severe arthritic pain and swelling.

OR!

Fresh, raw, mixed vegetable salad, including avocado pear, Icelandic prawns, parsley, Portuguese watercress, endives, enjoyed with a dash of healthy, zestful, absolutely pain free living?

If you are in pain and have arthritic swelling then I know which one you would chose. When I was in so much pain, had someone told me to go and eat grass I would have done so. You will not need much shelf space - that is where one stores tinned and packet food - foods that are designed to have a long shelf life and preserved accordingly. Beware! anything that has on the label **LONG LIFE**! You know what that means. It has been treated and preserved to have a long life and how on earth can that be natural or live food?

You will need refrigerator space for the 'alive' foods. Heads of lettuce (organic if possible), cauliflower, calabrese, spring greens, spinach (preferably raw), sprouts, organic cabbage, parsley, asparagus, beans, leeks, onions, (remember it is best to blanch these before cooking), any food or fruit that you have grown yourself or you have fresh and organic you can freeze down. Fruit is also included in this except strawberries! They contain massive amounts of histamine and often cause deleterious reactions.

YOU CAN ELIMINATE YOUR ARTHRITIC CONDITION IF YOU HAVE THE WILL!

If you have had extensive 'gold' or steroid treatment then you may have to be much more patient and even be prepared for the fact that it may not work for you at all. The irreversible damage done to blood platelets and the structural damage may well be too severe to rectify.

At one time, some years back now, if a patient booked in with an arthritic condition my Secretary was instructed to ask if they had been prescribed gold treatment; if the answer was in the affirmative I would not accept them. Then one day a couple came and the wife had been prescribed gold, so I asked them why they had kept the appointment. Quite rightly, the husband said, "what right have you to deny my wife the chance of getting better". I have no right to do so, my refusal was based on the fact that blood platelets had been irrevocably changed and I did not wish them to waste their time or money. "We are willing to try anything to get my wife better" he said, so I agreed to test her and warned that recovery could take much longer. "Were you warned that once taken they could have severe side effects?" I asked. "No" was the reply. It is amazing how few patients are. If you are a Doctor reading this please tell your patients that gold and steroid treatment is the last straw and the long term effects of these are not known.

As luck would have it she recovered in approximately six weeks, with diminishment of pain and swelling but, judged overall, her recovery was nothing like as quick as a patient who had not been prescribed gold. But, needless to say, from that day on I never refused a patient who had been prescribed gold and thankfully many have improved their quality of life considerably since that time. It is worth pointing out that should the worst scenario occur and you do not feel any major benefits, the diet and supplementation would still be worth doing to prevent any further deterioration. **Prevention is always better than cure**.

The real cause of arthritis is - (my hypothesis): -

1. The inability of the digestive system to tolerate certain foods - **pancreatic malfunction.**
2. A scarcity of the nutrients that the body requires . Supplementation required.
3. An overabundance of **chemical additives** used in the processing of foods, which our bodies do not need, and which indeed it cannot cope with.

You are not going to take bigger and better pills to cure your arthritis - simpler and for some worse than that - you are going to give up some of your favourite foods of a lifetime - a bitter pill indeed for some!!

YOU CAN ELIMINATE ARTHRITIS IF YOU HAVE THE WILL!

Here is a list of seventeen additives which will, in time, be proven to be harmful to the human system over a period of years.

1. BUTYLATED HYDROXYANISOLE - E 320.(BHA)
2. BUTYLATED HYDROXYTOLUENE -E 321 (BHT)
3. DISODIUM DIHYDROGEN PHOSPHATASE.

4. MONOSODIUM GLUTAMATE - SODIUM HYDROGEN L-GLUTAMATE E621.
5. CARAGEENAN - E407.
6. FOOD COLOURINGS.
7. SODIUM NITRATE - E 250/25 1.
8. SODIUM NITRITE.
9. POLYSORBATE 60- E 435.
10 POLYSORBATE 80- E 433.
11 DI-POTASSIUM PHOSPHATE - E 340(b).
12 SORBITAN-MONOSTEARATE - E 491.
13 OXYGEN INTERCEPTOR.
14 SULPHUR DIOXIDE - E 220.
15 BENZOATE OF SODA - E 211.
16 SODIUM SILICO ALUMINATE.
17 CARAMEL-E 150.

As recently as last week 08-09-2010 a programme on television was advising that there were safe e- numbers and that many of the products were natural. What was not pointed out was that if they were left in their natural state they would remain enzymatically acceptable, but they are then manufactured and the natural enzymes destroyed. Beware of false prophets!

Where possible I have added the E Numbers, which should enable you to use the 'Find Out' booklet available from Foresight and listed in useful addresses section in rear of book.

Now you are ready to start your treatment. Your body will love it. Your habit department will not. If you are a sufferer of osteo or rheumatoid arthritis the seven day programme will be the hardest, yet most rewarding, and important seven days of your life. There are many more case histories I could relate, but hopefully this one will give you heart and spur you on.

Mrs B.B. from "Nirvana" Weston-super-Mare relates her story as follows:"

In 1983 I began having severe pain and swelling throughout my body, also terrible mood swings - over the following three years my husband took me to three top specialists, who gave me every test imaginable to try and find out why I was so ill, also deteriorating so fast. On my last visit to a specialist I had got to the point where I was unable to work, either by being employed or working in my own home, i.e. housework etc. and relied heavily on my husband and family who would clean and cook for me, as it would take me at least three hours to mentally and physically get started in the mornings and some days even longer

The pain by now was becoming intolerable and even holding a cup became a mammoth task. After the specialist had examined me - he informed me there was nothing he could do for me, I had arthritis throughout my body - every joint and my ribs, and "I would have to live with it'. (Author. Note this typical reply!!). I was 47 at the time. On hearing this I discussed at home, my future, with my husband. I explained to him that that if I had to live with the rest of my life in such severe pain and so mentally slow - that I did not wish my life to continue - as the pain increased, my skin became unbearable to touch - so even a re-assuring cuddle was out of the question. I also realised the rate this debilitating disease was moving that within a year I would be unable to walk and would need a wheelchair.

A short while after this I was informed, by two different people, that a Mr Davies, who lived in Taunton, may be able to help me. By this time I was convinced there wasn't anyone who could help me, but decided to make an appointment to see him. So, in 1986 1 went along for my first appointment with Mr Davies. On arrival at the surgery we found Mr & Mrs Davies extremely understanding to my condition. In spite of this both my husband and myself were very dubious as to whether he could help me.

Mr Davies began the tests explaining everything to us, but then told me that, not only did I have arthritis, I also had 20 other things wrong with me, such as mastitis, severe headaches, heartburn, eczema etc.; so, although we politely listened to Mr Davies saying,"if I was to do exactly what he suggested then I would be cured in six weeks", we were just a little sceptical to say the least. (I would query this as I never say cure, but say that you should be feeling better, Author).

On returning home neither of us were completely convinced by what we had seen or heard - especially after consulting 'TOP' specialists in the past who could offer no help for my condition, and then, here was this man saying he could cure me, provided I stick by my 'new way of living' diet sheet. We talked it over for many hours and then decided I had nothing to lose - so lets try it, in the back of our minds we thought we would prove him wrong, as we could not possibly imagine how food could make me so ill.

The first three days were the most painful of my illness, and, although Mr Davies warned me I would feel worse, I never expected to feel so bad. I spent most of the three days in bed - eventually I was able to get up, and slowly over the next few weeks I began to feel better and at last able to have a full nights undisturbed sleep. After six weeks we returned for my second appointment with Mr Davies, I explained that I still had some arthritis in my thumb joints and ribs, he then checked me on all the other problems he had pointed out to me, and I found I only had three of them left. Mr Davies suggested that I kept a sample of all foods etc.; which passed through my mouth for the next two weeks and label them. This I did and at the end of two weeks I returned and Mr Davies checked out all the samples I had kept, ***eventually he found that my toothpaste was the culprit, as it had colouring in it.*** *Within two weeks of finding this out my life changed and since this time I have lived a pain free life (**unless I detract from the diet or eat a food I am allergic to**). I no longer have to rely on others to help me in any shape or form.*

Within a year of my last visit to Mr Davies I started my own catering business, before seeing him I would have never had the confidence to have done this. A few years ago I had reason to consult my doctors and mentioned to him that I had not seen him for five years, which was quite something, as when I was ill with arthritis I would see him weekly. I explained everything that happened to me during this time, but it was obvious ***he was not impressed - even when I pointed out that the proof was before his eyes.***

It is now thirteen years since I became a victim to arthritis. I have a very full life, I am four stone lighter, skin and hair 100% better. I look and feel ten years younger, but best of all I am now 'PAIN FREE'. Family and friends have been so impressed at the new me they have also consulted Mr Davies, not only with arthritis, but eczema, asthma, hiatus hernia - with equally wonderful results, and we shall continue to recommend Mr Davies to anyone who will listen because, without any doubt whatsoever, if Mr Davies had not been recommended to me I would not be here today to tell my story.

My husband and I would like to take this opportunity to say ***THANK YOU*** *Mr Davies for giving me back my life. We would be honoured if you would include my story in your book.*

Wishing you every good luck in the future.

I am delighted to say that 27 years later the first Christmas card we receive is always from this lady and her family. If you read this — **thank you!**

When I retired so many people asked me to keep in touch that I did postal consultations for four years. I do not carry out that procedure now. I was not sure that postal consultations were going to be of any value, how wrong I was. I had several patients in Verbier, Switzerland, I shall call them Mr & Mrs K, they had friends in Zimbabwe and the husband was in a very bad way with arthritis. In his own words heading for a wheelchair fast. The knees so badly affected that all sport was out of the question. As I was treating the husband the wife asked me to treat her too, although her condition was slightly different, I sent them a detailed questionnaire which they duly returned and from that and the symptomology they presented I was able to determine what the basic causatory 'triggers' may be. Together they started the special way of eating and I was delighted to receive a detailed report some six weeks later - they were both free of pain and improving in general health by the day in leaps and bounds. So my misgivings about postal consultations were soon laid to rest and I have to say many others have been treated since then with equal success, including friends of Mr & Mrs K in Zimbabwe. I have actually been in touch with Mrs K in the last week. I now have a web site www.gwynnedavies.com and patients are invited to make contact through this medium and I am still more than happy to help.

I really do not think I can add much to that. It portrays all the elements of everything I have endeavoured to explain to you. The first few weeks are very tough! You will have to grit your teeth and persevere, even at times when you feel you cannot endure any more. You may have to go in to great depth about what you are ingesting if things do not follow the correct path. You will find that if you detract from the diet you will get a reaction. This could, and I am sure will, be one of the best adventures of your life. To try varieties of fruit and vegetables not normally ingested. Getting to know the taste of good uncontaminated or non-processed food, perhaps for the first time in your life. You will be gladdened by your taste buds, for they will revel in the natural healthy taste of food. The one thought that must always be in the forefront of your mind is **BE POSITIVE**!!

So, gird your loins!! Pluck up courage!! Show what you are made of- and beat this dreaded disease for ever!!.

YOU DO NOT HAVE TO LIVE WITH ARTHRITIS IF YOU HAVE THE WILL!

Diet and Advice for Rheumatism and Arthritis

DAY ONE

Breakfast NONE
Lunch NONE
Dinner NONE

Drink at least four 8oz glasses of water.

Do not repeat. Continue with Day two and if still in pain after seven days then start again with day 2 and continue this until free of pain.

DAY TWO

start here if taking drugs, have fruit only on Day 1.

Breakfast Unsweetened grape or prune juice. Ripe banana.

Lunch Fresh lamb. Mixed green salad, oil and organic vinegar dressing.

(Not if on a candida diet, see separate diet for arthritis and candida).) Bowl of organic fruit in season.

Dinner Raw vegetable plate (Chinese leaves, celery, cucumber etc. Raw fruit salad (grated apples, pears, grapes, bananas etc. NO CITRUS 5m1 Flax Oil, or three full strength capsules, with a drink 2 hours after evening meal.. Try and make sure your fruit is ORGANIC. If not please make sure you peel all fruit.

DAY THREE

Breakfast Blended raw fruits. 4ozs boiled goat or sheep milk or soya (organic unsweetened) milk.

Lunch Fresh fillet of top fish lightly sautéed. Raw cauliflower or other raw vegetables. 4ozs boiled goat or sheep milk

Dinner Roast chicken, blanched onions or leeks, mixed green salad. Sautéed potato. Fresh fruit salad.

Flax Oil as for day two with a drink 2 hours after evening meal.

DAY FOUR

Breakfast Prunes or prune juice. Rice dream. 4ozs boiled goat or sheep milk.

Lunch Grilled lamb chops lightly sautéed. Mixed green salad. Basmati rice. Fresh fruit.

Dinner Halibut steak or other top fish steamed lightly. Mixed salad. Half avocado. Fruit in season.

Flax Oil as for previous nights with a drink 2 hours after evening meal.

DAY FIVE

Breakfast Fruit in season chopped up on puffed rice cereal.. Rice dream. 4ozs boiled goat or sheep milk.

Lunch Half avocado, sliced tomato, watercress, cress, spring onions. 4ozs boiled goat or sheep milk.

Dinner Roast duck or duckling, mixed green salad, Basmati rice. Fresh fruit. 4ozs goat or sheep milk.

Flax Oil as previous nights with drink 2 hours after evening meal.

DAY SIX

Breakfast Puffed rice, chopped fruit, rice dream.. 4ozs boiled goat or sheep milk.

Lunch Icelandic or Norwegian prawn salad. Cantaloupe or Ogan melon or fresh fruit. 4 ozs boiled goat or sheep milk.

Dinner Lightly grilled lamb chop, large chefs salad including raw peas, string beans, uncooked vegetables and greens. Plums or other raw fruit in season. 4ozs boiled goat or sheep milk.

Flax Oil as for previous nights 2 hours after evening meal.

DAY SEVEN

Breakfast Sliced bananas. 4ozs boiled goat or sheep milk.

Lunch Lightly broiled fish. Carrot sticks and watercress. Grapes. 4ozs boiled goat or sheep milk.

Dinner Lightly sautéed turkey, chicken etc; raw

vegetables mixed in blender. Honeydew melon or fruit in season(never strawberry). 4ozs boiled goat or sheep milk.

Flax Oil as for previous nights 2 hours after evening meal.

SPECIAL INSTRUCTIONS FOR ALL SEVEN DAYS

Take one B-Alive with each meal.

Drink only when thirsty, and then only juice of raw fresh fruit, or juice of raw fresh vegetables (organic whenever possible) or water bottled or filtered.(preferably a glass bottle) Goat or sheep milk will invariably be frozen; it is a full fat milk and you are advised to water this down to equal parts of 50%milk-50%water.

Substitute foods according to taste or season.

Continue this diet until pain and swelling disappear.

Add one food per day from the allowable list Appendix. A.

If after three weeks things are not improving as well as hoped then eliminate the B-Alive for a week and observe. If there is no change then re-introduce. Eliminate the blackstrap molasses for a week and observe. If there is no change then re-introduce. Watch carefully for any food that you may feel upsets you or increases the pain and eliminate that for a week. You really will be required to become a detective and the rewards will accrue.

Vegetarian options are better but if meat preferred then it must be organic.

Chapter 17

Foods to be watched

Non-whey fed pork - yes! Eggs - yes! Vegetarian or goat and sheep cheese - yes! **Remember**, do cook in oven to kill bacteria before eating. Only buy hard vegetarian cheeses and not red coloured cheeses.

You can add food after food to your permanent arthritis free life, one at a time every three days, so that you can spot a possible culprit. Those of you that have only been recently affected with arthritis can add foods faster than those suffering with long term damage and must give time to allow their joints to adjust. Having said that, **nobody** - I repeat **nobody** - should ever return to the hard core troublemakers that you have been warned about as allergens.

Foods That Must Always Be Watched Carefully

The more you avoid these items the safer you will be and the speedier will be your recovery.

1. Make sure you are free of pain, heat and swelling before introducing grains, porridge etc. Start with puffed rice and then organic white flour until you are absolutely sure there is no reaction; then you can introduce corn flakes and rice krispies (these contain sugar, so be careful) introduce brown flour slowly because it contains phytic acid and needs to be watched carefully.
2. All flour products like bread, toast, cakes(home baked with dairy free margarine), pizzas, pies, biscuits, crackers, doughnuts (contain milk), spaghetti, noodles etc. Once all pain and swelling has disappeared and you are sure that the organic white flour is acceptable with no reaction,

then you can gently add these products (except pizzas and doughnuts).

3. Coffee, tea, cocoa, liquor, beer, wine, coca or Pepsi cola, carbonated and soft drinks. After the first week you can introduce a good tea (not tea bags), such as Darjeeling, Assam or Luaka or Sencha green tea.
4. Sugars (always the biggest enemy even when organic) Swedish Glace ice cream.
5. Jellies, jams and marmalade. The exception to the rule here is if the fruit is organic and the minimum of organic sugar is used, then once free of pain they can be introduced slowly.
6. Tinned or processed foods, custards, puddings and prepared mixes.
7. Frozen fruits (unless they are organic).
8. Any food manufactured or adulterated by man, such as prepared breakfast cereals or semi-prepared ones like quick cooked oatmeal.

REMEMBER— 'LONG LIFE'- MEANS - PAINFUL LIFE!

Your Most Valuable Foods

Vegetables

Carrots, peas, black eyed peas, lima beans, string beans, runner beans, broad beans, French beans,corn, cucumber, marrow, courgette, cabbage, Savoy cabbage, calabrese, young leaf spinach, kale, kohlrabi, beet tops, parsnips, cauliflower, turnips, egg plant, broccoli, curly kale, Brussels sprouts, parsley, salsify, asparagus, onions, leek, chives, mushroom, brown rice, wild rice, lettuce, watercress, endive and beetroot.

FOWL

Free range chicken, duck, goose, pheasant, turkey, quail and pigeon.

MEATS

Now this is a tricky one with the past BSE scare, a tragedy really, as it is something I believe should never have happened. It is easy, as a vegetarian, to pass comment and be flippant, and say, 'Don't eat meat'. But an awful lot of people do eat it and enjoy it. Having given it a lot of thought, my advice would be this - if you are over the age of fifty the chances are it is too late anyway, so go ahead and eat beef, if you like it of course. It is the children that worry me and, if there is a genuine connection between BSE and Creutzfeld Jakob Disease, then children should not be fed beef or beef products unless it is guaranteed organic. Lamb and pork — should be non- whey fed and organically reared.

I do not advise any more the ingestion of organ meats (offal) or using the juices from the cooked meat. Use marmite (providing there is no candidiasis), Yeast free gravy mix or organic vegetable stock cubes from your health shop instead.

SEAFOOD

Bass, hake, bream, haddock (not smoked), cod, halibut, fresh salmon — (preferably not pellet fed), pollock, huss, gurnard and turbot.

FRUIT

Apples (always peeled unless organic), pears, banana, peach, plum, kiwi fruit, melon, blackberry, blueberry, raspberry, nectarines, apricots, grape and currants.

NUTS

Chinese chestnuts, walnuts, brazils, butternuts, cashews, almonds, pecans, peanuts (not *dry* roasted).

If you are a migraine sufferer then you are advised to check the citrus fruits individually and the nuts, as they can often be indicated. I would suggest that you become migraine free and then introduce one at a time and never more than two a week.

N.B. NOT HAZELNUTS.

SOUPS

Split pea, lentil, lima bean, pearl barley, leek and potato, tomato, mixed fresh vegetables etc.;

SEEDS

Sunflower, sesame, pumpkin, etc.;

EGGS

If you can obtain eggs that are definitely organic or free range then so much better.

CHEESES

Pecorino, Cabrales, Manchego, Feta, Chevres, Halumi, Eftaki and, often on your local market stalls or in health food shops, local goat or sheep's cheeses which are delicious. Remember cook in oven not grill to kill bacteria.

WARNING!

If you are a rheumatoid arthritic then you must not eat the following foods: - tomato, rhubarb, gooseberry, strawberry, beetroot, spinach, peppers or radish. Onion and leeks must be blanched before being put in the cooking by boiling for one minute and throwing the water away. Some people have to blanch the asparagus and celery too. It is always better to be safe than sorry!

It does not necessarily mean that these are banished forever. What often happens is that the basic allergy trigger is removed and items such as the above can then be introduced in small amounts without any ill effects. However, this does not mean eating a lot of any particular item; it really is a little and not too often.

Ten Commandments for Arthritis Free Dining

1. Balance your menu fairly evenly between proteins, fats and carbohydrates.
2. Eat some raw fruit or vegetable at every meal.
3. Avoid high heat cooking - it alters food structure and destroys nutrients. Frying with very low heat with a suitable oil to prevent food sticking to the pan is permissible. **Microwaves are total anathema** - DO NOT TOUCH! (Further information available from Coghill Research, Kermenez, Lower Race, Pontypool, Gwent, NP4 5UF).
4. Cook food as little as possible. Obviously in the winter months lightly cooked is the order of the day. Good home made soups etc.
5. Save vegetable juices produced in cooking. Use in soups, gravy, sauces etc or drink it.
6. Flesh and muscle meats are more suitable these days. Organ meats, unless certain they are organic, should be avoided if possible.
7. Favour whole natural food rather than extracts or parts of it. Eat the skin or outer covering where edible, not just the inside. This does not apply to apples or potato skin as the residual pesticides and sprays are lethal to us as arthritics. Peel them unless you can be sure they are organic. Apple juice should only be Meridian, Aspalls, Peakes, Prewetts, or Appleford (not in a carton either - bottles only please); they should be organic and marked as such.
8. Favour organic or natural sources of all meat and produce. The Soil Association do provide a booklet to subscribers; this lists suppliers of organic foods throughout the country.
9. Avoid entirely all flour and flour products in the early stages. Everyone is different but at least for six weeks in

most cases. Then introduce organic white flour first and ensure there is no reaction.

10. Thou shalt not commit adultery. Adulteration of foods we are talking about. There is a wonderful organisation called Foresight. Primarily set up many years ago as an organisation for the pre-conceptual care of women. The address will be in the useful addresses section at rear. They publish a superb little booklet called *Find Out,* this lists all the E Numbers in traffic light sequence: Red for danger - do not touch, Amber for caution - avoid if possible and Green for go (it is generally regarded as safe).

If you purchase this booklet you will be staggered at the amount of chemicals, additives and preservatives with which manufacturers adulterate our food. These are not really good for anyone who cares about their health but to us as arthritics they really are not permissible without paying a very real cost.

YOU DO NOT HAVE TO LIVE WITH ARTHRITIS!

SAFE FOODS

Organically reared beef, chicken or Iamb but, if not obtainable, then grill meat or cook on trivet.

Cod, coley, huss, haddock, halibut, pollack, whiting, bass, bream, hake, sea trout, turbot, Icelandic or Norwegian prawns.

Use organic vegetables whene ver possible. Chinese leaves are a safe salad alternative and Portuguese watercress.

DO WASH EVERYTHING WELL!

Malvern Evian, Volvic, Buxton, or Monastiere water etc.

Olive oil (cold pressed, first
pressing virgin oil is best),
linseed/flax oil, sunflower oil, safflower oil.

Ordinary plain potato crisps.

AVOID

Meat juices, meat fat, organ meats (liver, kidney etc), chicken skin and meat stock. Animals are injected with various drugs and this will avoid them.

Flatfish (plaice, dabs, flounder), shell fish (they feed on the sea bed which is heavily polluted), fish skin, coloured or smoked fish, mackerel, herring or pellet fed trout.

Watercress (absorbs nitrites), commercially sprayed lettuce, cucumber skin, potato skin, Dutch imported cabbage, red cabbage and outer leaves of commercially grown green vegetables.

Cherries (unless organic) and strawberry.

No carbonated waters.

No flavoured or low fat crisps.

Please remember these are guidelines. The whole way of eating is manoeuverable to suit the individual, particularly if you are a working person. Days can be changed round and meals can be changed round - as long as you keep to the basic tenets of the recommendations you will not go far wrong.

Microwaves

I referred earlier to not using microwaves for cooking. You the reader are bound to ask, "Why". Recent research shows that microwave oven-cooked food suffers severe molecular damage. When eaten, it causes abnormal changes in human blood and immune systems. Not surprisingly the public has been denied details on these significant health dangers. In 1989 an announcement sponsored by Young Families, the Minnesota Extension Service of the University of Minnesota stated,

> *"Although microwaves heat food quickly, they are not recommended for heating a baby's bottle. The bottle may seem cool to the touch, but the liquid inside may become extremely hot and could burn the baby's mouth and throat. Also the build up of steam in a closed*

> *container such as a baby's bottle could cause it to explode. Heating the bottle in a microwave can cause slight changes in the milk. In infant formulas there may be a loss of some vitamins. In expressed breast milk some protective properties may be destroyed. Warming a bottle by holding it under a hot tap or setting it in a bowl of hot water then testing it on your wrist before feeding may take a few minutes longer but is much safer".* (Valentine, Acres U.S.A. 1989).

You may well ask, "What have microwaves to do with arthritis?" They affect the immune system and, as already stated, an arthritic sufferer has a compromised immune system. Some years ago a young lad of thirteen was brought to me with rheumatoid arthritis; his joints were already distorted. Thankfully he recovered quite well after a few months and all went well for approximately nine months then out of the blue his condition began to worsen. His GP naturally said, "It is a regression; rheumatoid arthritics often 'flare' like this then it settles down again or burns itself out". I do not agree with that and I was anxious to find the causatory trigger. So he came back and we tested all his foods, his drinking water, his toothpaste - everything. We could find nothing. So, I said to the parents, the lad and his sister, "We must talk this through and find out what changed in the household at the time the condition worsened". After a few minutes Alistair said, "I know. It was when we bought the microwave". Needless to say, Mum and Dad agreed this was the case and the microwave was removed from the house and his condition improved immediately.

YOU DO NOT HAVE TO LIVE WITH ARTHRITIS!

Chapter 18

Food Irradiation

At the heart of a food irradiation plant stands a rack of 400 gamma ray emitting cobalt-60 rods. This highly radioactive source is housed in a concrete chamber with walls six feet thick. Food is placed in to the chamber to be irradiated.

According to the London Food Commission, properly used, the process does not create radioactive food but merely slows ripening (at low levels) or kills bacteria and pests (at high levels). The food can then be transported further around the world, left longer in the warehouse or on the shelf. (I cannot believe that the public are aware of this. 'Author' Waste is reduced. Profits increase and if you believe food irradiation supporters, nothing in the food changes chemically or nutritionally. Pigs might fly!!

It also increases the profits of the nuclear industry. The cobalt—60 rods are nuclear waste that would otherwise have to be held in special secure sites indefinitely.

Although irradiation can kill bacteria, it does not remove any toxins they have already produced and was actually found to increase aflatoxins, linked to liver cancer. This was found by three separate studies as far back as the 1970's.

Vitamins A,C,D,E and K and some B vitamins(1,2,3,6 and 12) are damaged by irradiation. The extent of the damage varies from food to food. Vitamins in fruit juice, for instance, are more vulnerable than in fresh fruit.

Irradiation converts nitrates to nitrites. **These are potent carcinogens.**

Pro-irradiation experts boast that irradiation reduces dangerous food additives (we are always being told these are safe) but, in fact, additives are added to irradiated food to control undesirable effects. Amongst these additives are sodium nitrite, sodium sulphite, potassium bromate, sodium triphosphate and glutathione.

The International Atomic Energy Authority, a keen supporter of irradiation, quotes several medical studies 'proving' the safety of irradiated foods. One study it appears to have missed is one published in the American Journal of Clinical Nutrition way back in 1975. Cited by cancer research specialist, George L. Trisch, in expert evidence given to a congressional hearing in 1987, it tells of an Indian trial using children with severe protein deficiency: 5 children were given non-irradiated wheat and 5 were given wheat irradiated 2-3 weeks earlier. After four weeks blood samples were taken. Those from the irradiated group contained gross chromosomal abnormalities. 2 weeks later another sample was taken. These showed a sharp increase in abnormal lymph cells. The trials were stopped immediately. The trials were then recommenced with wheat that had been irradiated 12 weeks earlier. This time it took six, rather than four weeks, for the abnormalities to appear. **The trial showed that irradiation had caused physical changes that, at least in malnourished children, had led to pre-cancerous cell production.**

This is ironic because (a) irradiation has been trumpeted as the solution to world hunger and (b) it has been adopted as the answer to safe food in many less industrially developed countries. The double irony is that many of these countries export irradiated ingredients to more industrially developed countries like the UK, where there is no obligation to list irradiated ingredients in processed foods. Currently, therefore, the only way to avoid irradiated food is to buy **organic** or locally produced foods. When you consider that this whole book has been written about ill patients and how necessary it is to eat sensibly and to create a healthy cellular structure, it makes nonsense of irradiation in its entirety. I do believe strongly that irradiated foods and ingredients should be marked clearly and allow the public to make that vital decision – **CHOICE!**

Many sanitary items are now increasingly being irradiated. These include medical disposable supplies, cotton balls, contact lens solution, feminine hygiene products and packaging materials. Then there's make-up, wine corks and cask bladders, beehives (minus the bees), bottles and plastic containers.

GM foods rear there ugly heads again because it is legal to put 0.9% GM content in food without putting it on the label, Beware of soya ingredients even in organic foods if not marked organic on the ingredients list e.g.; lecithin. The products that are mainly affected are maize and soya products, some tomatoes or potatoes. **BUY ORGANIC.**

Chapter 19

Things to remember

Make sure you refrigerate oils once they are opened.

Do not re-heat oils. Use once and dispose of it.

Avoid freezing ready cooked meals then re-heating them.

Avoid re-heating meals of any kind.

Fry or roast food with oils rather than margarine. Reserve these for cakes and pastries and eat them cold.

Avoid microwaved food entirely. It alters blood platelets within 15 minutes of ingestion whether it be cooked, thawed or refrigerated.

Use Non-Fluoride toothpaste. Boots have a very good one. There are also herbal toothpaste's without fluoride available in most Health Shops.

Avoid pasteurised goat or sheep milks where possible. The body does not cope easily with the altered state of the milk.

Avoid aluminium cookware if possible. Better to use stainless steel, glass, or enamel cookware.

Avoid overcooking food because carbon particles are deleterious.

You may well think I am being a bit over the top but I am only too aware of the problems we have had over the years and these are the things that have given the most cause for concern because, as arthritics, our immune systems are under threat and our reactions to toxins are heightened. Therefore it is prudent to be over cautious rather than under cautious.

Joint Repair

I have heard it said hundreds of times by patients, "Once the joints are damaged there is nothing that can be done about it".

This just is not true. If it was true then the left hip, I was told would need replacing by the time I was forty, would now have a prosthesis. It has not. In fact the X-rays show clearly that my hip is in a normal condition for a man of my age. I have in my possession many X-rays of patients before and after and bone scans too and they all show regeneration of bone after approximately twelve to eighteen months.

It is perfectly true to say that if no remedial steps are taken then regeneration of bone cannot take place. But we are talking about the people who take remedial steps and the advised supplementation; then, and only then, can regeneration take place. It really is up to you.

Exercise

This is another contentious area. There are those who recommend exercise and those who are vehemently against it. My experience is that with most things moderation is the keyword. By sitting around you are allowing calcification to take place and ligamenture and musculature to atrophy and you are then in a situation that if you do move around it is painful. It is therefore common sense to reach the halfway house with some exercise and some pain but do not exercise to the point where inflammation takes place.

Pain is nature's way of telling you something is not right and the sensible thing to do is listen to her. I recommend that for the first three weeks, whilst the body is learning to adapt to its new way of living and inflammation is going down, do not exercise. Once you are aware of easement of pain and inflammation - and the correlation I draw here is that you were unable to get out of bed in the morning without being incredibly stiff and the movements very limited and then one morning you wake up, swing the legs out of bed and proceed to the bathroom without pain and stiffness - then it is time to think about gentle exercise.

After all, what you are trying to achieve slowly but surely is a return to normality but you must learn to walk before you can run. Some years ago I thought I was better so off I went to the golf course thinking I was going to play a round of golf. After three holes I was very glad to come home again. Another case comes to mind where a patient I had seen three months previously, who had made excellent progress in that time, presented with swollen hands and wrists and fingers like little puffed up sausages. I asked the obvious question, "Have you deviated from the diet?" and the answer was, "No. The only thing I have done out of the ordinary was two days ago I was feeling so much better that I pruned a few roses". I then asked, as this should not have caused that much swelling, "How many roses did you prune?" The answer she gave solved the problem immediately. "Oh! I suppose there must be forty eight rose bushes". Had she pruned only four there is every chance that the hands would have remained normal.

Bones repair very easily but ligaments, tendons and muscles take a lot longer and it is these that you have to gently encourage back to normal usage. It is more than likely that if there has been distortion of joints then repair will take time. One of the gentlest and painless ways of recovery is hydrotherapy - swimming. Having the support of the water is advantageous but it also slows movements down and prevents damage. When sitting in the evenings watching television, a good exercise for the hands is a medium tension squash ball squeezed gently but firmly for a dozen times in each hand, left for an hour or two and repeated. Again, in moderation please. Do not overdo it and the temptation is always there. If the hands are very sore next day - then you have exceeded your own capabilities - cut back!

A good exercise, if the feet are affected, is to get the old fashioned toilet roll holder with a wooden centre, take this out and, when sitting in the evenings, roll this under the ball of the foot backwards and forwards in a gentle rocking movement. The same thing applies if very sore next day - cut back!

As the condition improves and walking is possible then this is a wonderful gentle form of exercise too. Always start on level ground and make it a short walk to start with and gradually build up. The one thing not to do if the knees are affected is knee bends. To exercise knees you must lie on your back, bend the legs and grasping hold of the ankles gently pull them toward you and then release. Do this three or four times to start with and gradually build up.

If any of you have suffered from Halix Rigidus (the big toe becomes very stiff and a bunion starts to form) then you must gently but firmly exercise that joint by pulling the toe downwards and upwards. You may well hear grinding noises but this is nothing to worry about. As each day moves on you will find movement is increased and walking more comfortable. A gentle pull and push in the lateral plane is also of value. As the joint eases you will be able to rotate the toe quite easily.

If you have a knee problem and in some patients both knees are severely swollen, then it is possible that, after the first fortnight to three weeks, the swelling will go down and the

pain will ease; then some days later the pain returns. This inevitably means that the calcus formation has been broken down but the cartilage, tendons and musculature are learning to adapt to their new environment and, being used more than normal, inflame. Ice packs wrapped in a tea towel and applied for ten to fifteen minutes twice daily often help this condition. Should the condition persist, then have an X-ray and you and your practitioner will know what to do for the best.

Constipation

It really is quite amazing how many patients report this as a life long problem. Some actually report that it is common for them to only go once a week. I need not tell you that this is not normal and certainly will not be allowable. It is essential, as far as I am concerned, that you pass a motion at least once daily - preferably twice.

One thing I would not wish you to do is to take Senokot or any other purgative. There are various aids to help with this problem. The one that seems to suit everybody is Linusit Gold from your local health shop. Herbilax is another. The most natural way is with magnesium ascorbate - Vitamin C. This is in capsule or powder form and is available from Biocare Ltd (Tel:0121 433 3727). This can be taken without any side effects until the stool is loose. If it turns to diarrhoea then cut back slightly. On the first day take one teaspoon in organic juice or water morning and night. If no motion the following morning then add a further teaspoon at lunch time and continue increasing by a teaspoon each day until relief is obtained. A teaspoon is equivalent to 4 grams so if you are taking tablets equate the dosage. You may find that, after being on the Arthritic way of eating for three weeks, the bowel settles down and no problems are encountered. Should the problem continue then consult your practitioner as there are tests that can be carried out to ascertain the problem. As a precaution drink 2 glasses of filtered water before breakfast.

When Can I?

The question that arises with every patient, and it is a difficult one to answer.

When can I introduce bread? This, inevitably, is the first question ever asked and the most difficult one to answer. There are varying opinions on why the grains have such an effect on our systems, from the build up of residual pesticides, which remain in the endosperm even after grading, and the fact that many arthritics cannot tolerate and break down the husk and the bran in whole-wheat flour and produce phytic acid. This then produces stiffness and pain. So, the answer really is very much a trial situation. I suggest the following to my patients. Introduce white bread and see if there is a reaction after a week or two.

Thankfully the numerous additives and preservatives in white flour have now been removed but I must stress at this point that I am referring to plain white flour as many self raising flours have various reactive agents in them.

If all is well, and you are free of pain, then, and only then, introduce the whole grains, whole-wheat, porridge, barley etc. If you notice an increase in swelling, inflammation or pain, then stop immediately. It is far better to alternate for a few weeks until the system acclimatises and learns to cope. It is never a good idea to have anything on a daily basis.

When can I introduce coffee? The answer is simple really, **"Never"**. The reactions that take place when coffee is drunk should be enough to put anyone off. As mentioned earlier in the book, reiterated here to drive the point home, the comments usually passed are that the after effects were not worth the ingestion. This is what happens when you drink two cups of coffee:

Within a few minutes the temperature of the stomach jumps 10-15 degrees F.

There is an increase of up to 400% in its secretion of hydrochloric acid.

Your salivary glands double their output and your heart beats 15% harder.

Blood vessels get narrower in and around the heart.

Your metabolic rate goes up by 25% and your kidneys excrete 100% more urine.

Apart from these, ingesting this substance leads to hypoglycaemia, (which is opposite to diabetes) and eventual breakdown of the pancreatic system. Do you still want a coffee? I doubt it.

When can I introduce alcohol?

The answer here is as straightforward as for grain - when free of pain and swelling. When you are sure that you are well on the road to recovery then, as with the grains, introduce very gently and observe very carefully for any niggles or fleeting pains occurring or even swelling. If you are clear then you are certainly advised to have real ales, brewed correctly without the use of chemicals. Guinness is an example. If you have a dairy intolerance then you would not go for a milk-stout such as Mackesons or Baileys cream sherry etc. Try good quality white wine above Kabinett level; the price should tell you whether it is good or not. Chateau bottled red wines are worth trying but do make sure there are no reactions. You can try gin (but not the tonic), whisky of good quality, and vodka but, if you are rheumatoid, not the Bloody Mary.

I must stress, because it is so important, no matter how much you may like it, you must not commence alcohol until you are positive of real improvement and watch very carefully for adverse reactions. The biggest problem with alcohol is finding the appropriate mixer such as tonic water, which, like most of them, has chemicals and additives in them that are best avoided. Soda water is all right so whisky and soda is fine but gin and soda? - Not really. Several patients have told me they water down their drinks with water quite successfully, including wine. It really is a matter of trial and error and I would say the report back situation, regarding the intake of alcohol, is 50-50. So take care - proceed cautiously and ensure that you are not kidding yourself! In cheating you are only cheating one person – **YOU! REMEMBER IT IS SAFER TO LEAVE ALCOHOL ALONE COMPLETELY!**

Mrs J.P.L. Backwell. Bristol.

Dear Mr Davies

Gradually I noticed that my fingers were swollen at times and then they became painful. As it was during the winter of 1991/2 I was not unduly surprised. Then walking became painful — my knees ached and it was a struggle to walk our elderly dog and for me to use the motor mower to cut the lawns. I avoided bending down when possible. My hands became so awkward that I had difficulty in doing up buttons, using the controls for the washing machine and the dishwasher, unscrew trig bottle caps and threading a needle with sewing cotton. I had difficulty driving my car because of the pain in my knees and the inability to turn my head sufficiently to see through the rear windscreen when reversing.

At times writing was difficult and painful. I was tired and everything seemed an effort. I found that the pain in my hands kept me awake in the early hours of the morning and could not get comfortable. Being on a diet to prevent sinusitis (recommended by Gwynne Davies), I was not keen to take any painkillers. I was worried about the future for my family and myself — fearing that I would lose the ability to do things for them and myself

Someone suggested that I had arthritis and recommended that I took cod liver oil. I did this but the arthritis was so painful that I decided to seek medical help and visited my GP in February 1992. My doctor looked at my swollen hands, noticed the lack of mobility and listened to my complaint of pain — especially in the early hours of the morning A blood test was taken and the result indicated that I was suffering from osteo-arthritis on a diet to prevent sinusitis (recommended by Gwynne Davies), I was not keen to take any painkillers. I was worried about the future for my family and myself — fearing that I would lose the ability to do things for them and myself

Someone suggested that I had arthritis and recommended that I took cod liver oil. I did this but the arthritis was so painful that I decided to seek medical help and visited my GP in February 1992. My doctor looked at my swollen hands, noticed the lack of mobility and listened to my complaint of pain — especially in the early hours of the morning A blood test was taken and the result indicated that I was suffering from osteo-arthritis

In March 1992 1 visited Gwynne Davies who diagnosed candida albicans as a contributory factor to the osteo-arthritis.

He prescribed a diet to combat the candida albicans and arthritis together with courses of varying lengths of time of calcium caprylate (MycopryD, magnesium ascorbate l/it C), Uritol together with sulphur and Aesculus (to overcome constipation which I had for a very short time), Bioacidophilus (changed to Vegedophilus), B-Alive, NAG (N-Acetyl Glucosamine) and Eradicidin. I now take one multi-vitamin tablet, one Vegedophilus capsule, three B-Alive tablets, three NAG and six cod liver oil capsules daily.

I have not taken any painkillers nor any antibiotic tablets since seeing Gwynne Davies about my sinusitis in December 1989 (nearly six years ago).

Apart from a bad reaction I had one day, which I think was due to die back of candida albicans and a spell of constipation, I have enjoyed excellent health. I have fewer colds than before, no sinusitis, athlete's foot is a thing of the past, sore throats are minimal, scratches and cuts heal quickly and without festering, mouth ulcers (which used to be a problem) are rare, soreness inside my nostrils has gone and I am fitter than have ever been. Having a sugar free diet has resulted in only one small filling in a tooth in six years. My little fingers have enlarged joints and only hurt when I bend them severely. Otherwise, I lead an active life and can do anything that I want to do e.g. gardening, driving, sewing, walking and writing without any difficulty. I am free of pain! Only very occasionally I get a little stiffness but it soon wears off.

For a while I was worried by the grinding of some of my joints e.g. in my neck when turning my head and in my knees when walking upstairs. NAG and B-Alive have probably helped here. Since increasing the dosage the problem has reduced so that I am rarely aware of it now

When my arthritis was bad, I did not think it would be possible to ever have another dog in the future. After Gwynne Davies's treatment and the resulting improvement in my health, my husband and I bought a Border Collie puppy in July 1992. She is now fully grown with boundless energy and we walk miles together over varied terrains in all weathers. I take her to agility classes and run around the course with her without any difficulty.

At 59 years of age, as a private tutor and Parish Councillor, I lead a full and active life. It involves among other things taking on responsibilities, making and keeping appointments together with resolving problems caused by other people. I find that stress makes me want to eat and I probably have too many snacks. Sometimes my hands are a little swollen and I consider that to be stress related. I keep strictly to the diet recommended by Gwynne Davies.

Having suffered arthritis, I appreciate now being able to do all the things again that were once taken for granted. This has probably resulted in cramming too much into each day without taking time for relaxation.

I am most grateful to Gwynne Davies for all his advice and help which has resulted in restoring me to good health.J.P.L.

Miss.R.D. Chard. Somerset.

Little did I imagine that the early part 1981 would herald for me an experience which directed my journey in life on a totally new path. For several years I had been coping with arthritis which mainly affected my right knee and hands. Pain and stiffness increased and I consulted my GP who prescribed Opren (which constipated me) and arranged for an appointment with an Orthopaedic surgeon.

As months progressed ,I needed a walking stick to get about and my fingers were so painful and swollen, that simple actions like buttoning a blouse, holding a pen to write, turning a handle or gripping the wheel of my car, all proved intensely uncomfortable and often tears of frustration overcame me.

The consultant surgeon assured me that in due course I qualify for a knee replacement! Upon hearing this my innermost being soared into a determined, "you are not replacing anything of mine". Months passed and I felt worse plus feeling aged, immobile and doomed.

One day a friend suggested that I consult Mr Davies in Taunton. Mid March 1981, my consultation with Mr Davies took place. After some detailed testing for foods which were likely to aggravate my condition, I was advised to eliminate from my diet foods like — dairy products stimulants such as coffee, tea, chocolate, alcohol, acid forming foods like tomato, rhubarb, strawberries, oranges, additives, flavourings and colourings and above all, wheat flour.

I shall never forget that after advising me about my diet and what supplements to take, Mr Davies stated you do not have to live with arthritis for the rest of your life, but there is *nothing more I can do for you ". I felt shocked and shattered my hopes for relief from pain annihilated. Then Mr Davies added, 'YOU have to do it for yourself'.*

Earnestly I embarked on my diet and, in a few weeks I felt much worse. Colleagues at work urged me to "get off this crazy diet". I felt very disheartened but was determined to persevere.

After three weeks with no improvement, I phoned Mr Davies and explained how I felt. To my astonishment Mr Davies said, "Yes, that all sounds very good to me, it is the toxins leaving your system — please persevere . And, so I did. Another three and a half weeks later after my floor exercises to ease my stiffness, I realised that I got up from the floor with increased mobility, which allowed me to bend my knees and move my hands freely. I wanted to run around the neighbourhood shouting, "Look at me, I can move and run ". I was elated and phoned Mr Davies to give him my good news.

Sharing one's euphoria can be all the more poignant, especially when an individual wills the triumph over the odds for another. Mr Davies was just such a person for me. I know that my diet is a lifetime commitment, but the benefits of mobility, good health and vitality are rewards in themselves. These qualities have enhanced my whole being physically, mentally, spiritually and contributed to my change of career into Complimentary Therapies. Rare blessings do happen on life's journey and I shall always give thanks for Mr

Davies's intervention in my healing process.
R.D.

Arthritis and Candida

Talking about arthritis and candida is a good lead into warning you about the link between arthritis and candida. First of all what is candida? In the simplest of terms it is a proliferation of yeast in the gut that has created an alkaline/acid imbalance. The candida albicans being the stronger takes over and eliminates the healthy bacteria. Forgive me for reiterating this piece on candida/ parasitosis but there will be people who purchase this book and, being impatient to get better will go straight to the chapter on arthritis and possibly read the rest later, so it is for the "dippers" that this is aimed at.

Because of the imbalance, the mucosal lining of the gut is depleted and becomes permeable, then the mycellae enter into the blood and lymphatic system and become "systemic". Because it is an umbrella term it is difficult to determine which of the enormous group of parasites is responsible. Certainly the most common where arthritis is concerned is ***Endolimax Nana*** which can cause reactive arthritis and a great deal of pain. Certainly where rheumatoid arthritis is concerned. If treated properly this can be eradicated but needs to be under the guidance of a qualified practitioner.

Is there a way of recognising the symptoms of Candida? Yes!

An abnormally bloated stomach is one common symptom.
General feeling of being bloated is another.
Thrush in the throat or vagina.
Athletes foot.
Anal irritation.
Sudden onset of moles or warts.

These are the most obvious symptoms to watch out for but

there are others which, under normal circumstances, you would not associate with candidiasis.

Depression, irritability, anxiety neuroses.

Allergies fatigue.

PMT, menstrual problems, intermittent bleeding, hormonal instability.

Asthma, cravings for sugar, bread, alcohol.

Joint swellings and arthritis.

It can be the opinion of many of the medical profession that, if you do not have oral or vaginal thrush, you do not have candida. I would disagree with this totally. My experience over the last twenty years is that any of the above symptoms can be a pointer to the condition and should not be ignored. To ignore these symptoms is to allow a pre-disposing condition to remain a causatory factor, thereby lessening the chances of a full or even partial recovery.

The secret of finding the cause of arthritis is to follow the logical steps I have written down for you. If in doubt contact your practitioner.

When I wrote my last book it was the 28th August, 1996. The day I retired from full practice, I had seen my last patient and I have to say it was with very mixed feelings as no Immunologist had been appointed at Musgrove Hospital, Taunton, and I was the last allergy expert in Taunton in private practice., However I could look forward to writing and helping people that way. It is now November 2010 and I have not stopped helping patients or teaching students since that day either on the internet or by post and now of course writing this book. If any of you need help I suggest you tab in to my web site www.gwynne.h.davies.com and get in touch.

However, on that day, which I feel is very appropriate; I received the following letter from

Mrs S of Torquay.

Dear Mr Davies,

Thank you for your letter and the questionnaire on arthritis which I have answered as best I can - I hope it will assist you in writing your book – of course I have no objection at all in my name being used - I cannot sing your praises enough, you know that. How anybody medical or otherwise can dispute what you have done for arthritics is beyond me. I can only say they have never suffered the pain or they would change their minds - it is so absurd - I for one am the living proof of the wonder of allergens and the exclusion diet - and it doesn't cost expensive treatments or the threat of hip replacements and the horror of surgery.

I must admit that I came to you doubting as I have little time for general medicine - being a trained nurse of the old school makes me that way - my sister Gillian made the appointment for me to see you as she was upset to see me as I was, and what a difference you have made to my life and I am sure hundreds more - may your good work carry on through your books.

I wonder if you are retiring this month as you said you were when I last saw you. I shall miss you very much even if I don't need to see you was a comfort to know you were not far away.

If I can be of any further help to you please let me know - meanwhile the very best of luck to you and your wife, and may you write a best seller and make a fortune.

Best wishes to you both.

22nd August 1996.

YOU DO NOT HAVE TO LIVE WITH ARTHRITIS!!

Funny really, I do miss my patients very much, and new challenges always await but two patients said on that last day, "We shall miss you being there as a crutch". [have never been called that before but I think I know what they mean. It is always a comfort to know your practitioner, who you have known and trusted for years, is there when you need a shoulder to cry on or a helping hand when in trouble, and, as one of my patients kindly described me, the rock. If I have been that then I am pleased and grateful. Also very humble that I was given the opportunity late in life to re-train and help so many patients to lead a new and healthy life - a little bit different from the rather stressful life as an Air Traffic Controller in the Fleet Air Arm. To all of you who read this book, I thank you for reading it and I thank you my patients from the bottom of my heart - you have encouraged me and made me so determined to tell you through writing that with determination and application -

YOU DO NOT RAVE TO LIVE WITH ARTHRITIS!!!

Vis Medicatrix Naturae - Hippocrates.(The healing power of Nature).

May I add a postscript because it does say everything you need to know as an arthritic. On Christmas Eve 15 months ago Rosemarie and I paid our annual visit to Norman & Lil, two old farming friends of my dear father in law. I was appalled to see that Norman was absolutely crippled with rheumatoid arthritis. The swellings of his ankles, knees and hands were gross and he was near to tears as his pain was so severe. I asked him what he had done about it and of course he had been to his GP and been given painkillers and steroids; these were in addition to the Losec he had been on for many years. I asked him if he would like help and he *was* receptive to that. I tested him and found that he was hypersensitive to dairy produce and the tomato, rhubarb etc group of foods.

He went through the withdrawal phase and the swellings and pain subsided but he was never as good as I thought he should be. We then found he was allergic to lactose and the medication he was taking contained this. So we removed them. Things improved that bit more but something was missing. Fortunately his son had been watching a programme on TV about lactose intolerance. He suggested that father should stop the goat milk he was on as this was also lactose. I had overlooked that and felt very guilty about the months lost because of that slip of memory.

However he progressed normally but the thing that was now prominent in his symptomology was excessive urination at night so there was still something not right. He kindly gave us some big onions he had grown in his garden. They upset us both very badly so we asked Norman to bring some in for testing – positive reaction! Tested him on a normal onion – negative reaction! What on earth could there be in onion that was so bad? It was then that Rosemarie asked him what he had used on the plot the previous spring - cow manure from his pal down the road. Nitrites? Antibiotics? His swelling of joints is now down to normal, the knees are back to normal, the hands are nearly normal and his ankles and feet are almost there.

Whatever the reason, it taught Norman and me a lesson and one that I would like to pass on to you. It was a salutary lesson to me and one that to this day 'keeps me on my toes'.

Pain is nature's way of telling you something is wrong! So, if you have done the diet and still have pain or swelling then look for the causatory 'trigger'. I wonder where you have heard that before?

I would like to finish this chapter with a poem that applies not only to practitioners but also to any patient who takes up 'the challenge.'

THE PIONEERS

We shall not travel by the road we make;
Ere day by day the sound of many feet
Is heard upon the stones that now we break,
We shall come to where the crossroads meet.
For us, the heat by day, the cold by night,
The inch slow progress, and the heavy load,
And death at last to close the long grim fight,
With man and beast and stone, for them the road!

For them the shade of trees that now we plant,
For safe, smooth journey and the final goal,
Yea, birthright in the Land of Covenant –
For us, day labour, travail of the soul.
And yet the road is ours, as never theirs!
Is not one joy on us alone bestowed?
For us, the master: Joy, 0 Pioneers:
We shall not travel, but we make the road.
Anonymous.

Chapter 20

Strokes/Ischaemia

A sudden attack of weakness affecting one side of the body. It is the consequence of an interruption of the blood flow to the brain. The primary disease is in the heart or blood vessels and the effect on the brain is secondary. The flow of blood may be prevented by clotting (thrombosis), a detached clot that lodges in an artery (embolus), or rupture of an artery wall (haemorrhage),. A stroke can vary in intensity from a passing weakness or tingling in a limb to a profound paralysis, coma and death.

Ischaemia

An inadequate flow of blood to a part of the body, caused by constriction or blockage of the blood vessels supplying it. Ischaemia of heart muscle produce ***angina pectoris.*** Affecting the brain ***cerebral haemhorrage.***

Strokes are not pleasant and an associated condition is Bells Palsy where the muscles in the side of the face collapse and droop. For many years now I have treated very successfully patients suffering from these conditions. The sooner help can be given the more dramatic the recovery. It is a homoeopathic preparation called Convallaria 30 tincture 10 ml dropper, place 5 drops under the tongue, wait 5 minutes and repeat5, wait a further five minutes and repeat again. You should see a response quite quickly. I will give you an example –

Just after I retired from practice we received a call from a very dear Italian friend in a mumbling and almost incoherent speech pattern saying "I think I have had a stroke". Stay there said I, will be with you in a few minutes. Five minutes later we were at her house and it was obvious she had indeed had a stroke, she could not speak properly, her right arm was limp, she could not stick her tongue out, so I put 5 drops of Convallaria under tongue, waited and repeated 3 times, half an hour later she was able to converse normally and could write her own name clearly. A perfect example of the wonders of homoeopathy correctly prescribed.

The simple way is to remember it as plaque building up on the walls of the arteries and therefore creating a narrowing and in some cases producing a clot. That in turn reminds me of a story told to me many years ago by Mary Tomlinson and introduces a sense of humour in to what is a serious subject. I hope you will have a chuckle.

LORD THROMBOSIS

A story told to Richard Tomlinson many years ago by Henry Plumb (Lord Plumb's) father.

Aneurin Bevan was being a nuisance in the House Of Commons, They wished to be rid of him, so, they offered him a Life Peerage.

"On leaving the House that day he met Winston Churchill, who asked him what title he would be taking. Nye Bevan said he did not really know and would have to think about it.

Winston said What about Lord Thrombosis?

Nye Oh! Yes! I like that, it sounds well. Lord and Lady Thrombosis, I shall have to see Jenny and see what she thinks.

He got home and told Jenny about meeting Winston outside the House and *his* suggestion of Lord and Lady Thrombosis. Jenny said she liked it but she said I don't trust Winston I think it means something. So, she took the dictionary from the library shelf and looked up the word thrombosis only to find that it meant

"A bloody clot which *is* difficult to remove"

Chapter 21

Heart disease

Heart Surgeon Admits Huge Mistake

Now we get on to the serious business of arterial /inflammation by Dr Dwight Lundell MD. CV at end of article. Read it carefully and then I will tell you the ten deadly foods.

During my 25 years as a cardiac surgeon, along with other prominent physicians labelled "opinion makers," we insisted heart disease resulted from the simple fact of elevated blood cholesterol. The only accepted therapy was prescribing medications to lower cholesterol and a diet that severely restricted fat intake.

Pharmaceutical giants reported $33 Billion dollars in cholesterol lowering drugs last year. As a nation, we reduced the fat content in our diets faithfully and yet with 25% of the population taking statin medications, more Americans will die this year of heart disease than ever before and at a younger age.

Don't you think something is terribly wrong?

Let me say those traditional recommendations are no longer scientifically or morally defensible; in fact, the consequences dwarf any historical plague in terms of mortality, human suffering and dire economic consequences.

Statistics from the American Heart Association show that ***75 million Americans currently suffer from heart disease, 20 million have diabetes and 57 million have pre-diabetes****. These disorders are affecting younger people in greater numbers every year.*

Low-fat diet recommendations with elimination of saturated fat are responsible for epidemics in inflammation, heart disease, obesity and diabetes. Let's look at why:

Hidden Omega-6 Oils

Processed foods are manufactured with Omega-6 oils for longer shelf life; chips and fries are soaked in soybean oil. Omega-6's are essential as they are part of every cell membrane controlling what goes in and out of the cell but without a correct balance to Omega-3's, more harm sets in.

If the balance shifts to excessive Omega-6, the cell membrane produces chemicals called cytokines that directly cause inflammation. Today's main stream diet has produced an imbalance from 15:1 to as high as 30:1 in favor of Omega-6. That's a tremendous amount of cytokines causing inflammation. A ratio of 3:1 would be optimal and healthy.

Animal fats contain less than 20% Omega-6 and are much less likely to cause inflammation than the supposedly healthy oils labelled polyunsaturated. The science that saturated fat alone causes heart disease is non-existent. The science that saturated fat raises blood cholesterol is also very weak.

Perfect Brain and Memory Health

Imagine how great it will feel to enjoy life without the fear, embarrassment, or frustration of mental slip-ups. You won't have to worry about forgetting people's names... or missing appointments... or misplacing your glasses...or locking yourself out of your car or house.

Read on to find out more...

Add Harm From Sugars and Simple Carbohydrates

Simple carbohydrates and refined sugars cause the body to produce high levels of insulin from the pancreas. Over time, cells will become sensitive and less resistant to excessive insulin creating Type 2 diabetes. Then they become abnormally stiff from an overload of Omega-6 fatty acids.

When we consume more sugars than we use or need, ***a cycle of internal terror begins*** *as our bodies are not designed to eliminate toxic substances. Cells will become overloaded producing a substance* *called resistin that makes cells even less responsive to insulin.*

LDL is chemically changed from this cycle of internal terror becoming abnormal. The LDL chemical changes are perceived by the body as an invader, an infection or foreign substance to be destroyed and the inflammatory process begins.

The important point to remember is ***LDL would not become trapped in the artery wall and cause a plaque*** *unless the LDL changed from oxidation or high blood sugar in the presence of inflammation.*

Without inflammation being present, cholesterol would move freely throughout as nature intended.

What About Weight?

Excess weight creates overloaded fat cells that pour out large quantities of pro-inflammatory chemicals that add to the injury caused by having high blood sugar. In time this vicious cycle creates heart disease, high blood pressure, diabetes and finally, Alzheimer's disease, as the inflammatory process continues unabated.

Arterial Inflammation

Inflammation is simply your body's natural defense to a foreign invader such as a bacteria, toxin or virus. The cycle of inflammation is perfect in how it protects your body from bacterial and viral invaders. However, if we chronically expose the body to injury by toxins or foods the human body was never designed to process, a condition results called chronic inflammation.

Chronic inflammation is just as harmful as acute inflammation is beneficial.

I have seen inside thousands upon thousands of arteries. Arterial inflammation (diseased artery) looks as if someone took a brush and scrubbed repeatedly against its wall. Several times a day, every day, the foods we eat create small injuries compounding into more injuries, causing the body to respond continuously and appropriately with inflammation.

What's the Answer to This Fire Raging in Our Bodies?

It's not as difficult as you might think. Return to foods closer to their natural state. If a food is packaged and processed or labelled "low-fat or no-fat diet" it is high in sugar or high in Omega-6 oil. Check a few packages and you'll see soybean oil as a major ingredient.

Choose carbohydrates that are very complex such as colorful fruits and vegetables. Cut down on or eliminate inflammation-causing Omega-6 fats. One tablespoon of corn oil contains 7,280 mg of Omega-6; soybean contains 6,940 mg. Instead, use olive oil or butter from grass-fed beef.

You can reverse inflammation in your arteries and throughout your body from consuming the typical American diet by following my recommendations in The Great Cholesterol Lie. You'll learn essential vitamins and minerals to add, inflammatory foods to eliminate, how to eat safely in fast food chains and a list of recommended tests to measure your risk factor for heart disease.

This is neither complicated nor mysterious yet conflicting information abounds making it appear so. Death happens only once but good health is a continuum.

Editor's Note: *Dr. Dwight Lundell is the past Chief of Staff and Chief of Surgery at Banner Heart Hospital, Mesa, AZ. He is the founder of Healthy Humans Foundation and Chief Medical Advisor for Asantae. In 2003, Dr. Lundell made the most difficult decision of his 25 year surgical career. As traditional medicine continued to chase the cholesterol theory of heart disease, Dr. Lundell closed his surgical practice. He then devoted the rest of his life to speaking the truth that inflammation causes heart disease. By lowering inflammation, heart disease has a cure.*

Dr. Lundell is the author of the world-wide bestselling book, The Great Cholesterol Lie.This book is a revealing look at heart disease and the faulty theories of low-fat diets and cholesterol. He also reveals his clinically-tested recommendations for lowering inflammation that can prevent and reverse heart disease. ***Click here now to learn more.***

Poison in Your Grocer's Produce Section

Clean food activists have discovered that 12 common fruits and vegetables - when conventionally grown - are absolutely TOXIC. The "Dirty Dozen" have been raised with so many pesticides there's no way to wash them off. Even peeling these fruits and vegetables will not rid them of the toxins.

This "horror list" includes all-time favorites like apples and spinach… Plus 10 others that most of us eat regularly.

If you wish to learn more about Dr Lundell then go on to the internet as I did and download the information therein.

Which foods is he referring to.

What Should You Buy Organic?

The 43 different fruit and vegetable categories listed for over 43,00 different pesticides these 12 fruits and vegetables had the **highest pesticide** load, making them the most important to buy or sow organic.

Peaches
Apples
Sweet bell peppers
Celery
Nectarines
Strawberries
Cherries
Lettuce
Grapes
Pears
Spinach
Potatoes

The following twelve had the **lowest pesticide** load when conventionally grown. Consequently they are the safest non organic crops to eat.

Broccoli

Aubergine
cabbage
Banana
Kiwi
Asparagus
Peas (frozen)
Mango
Pineapple
Sweet corn (frozen)
Avocado
Onion

Once again this points out to us how important it is to **GO ORGANIC.**

Needless to say throughout my practice life and since I have had to deal with many patients with heart disease and in each case once they were tested the most common sensitivity was to milk and dairy products in toto. As Dr Lundell states clearly the elimination of these in themselves will not be enough in isolation. That is why I always put patients on the elimination of toxins diet and recommended a healthy meat and fat reduced diet for the rest of their lives.

Keeping up to date with trends and information. Now in November 2010 an advert in a national newspaper for Cardiac Risk in the Young (CRY). **EVERY WEEK AT LEAST 12 APPARENTLY FIT AND HEALTHY YOUNG PEOPLE IN THE UK DIE FROM UNDIAGNOSED HEART CONDITIONS. Tel; 01737 363222.** A wake up call? I think so.

Now we get to the most important statement I will ever make with regard to heart conditions, high blood pressure etc; If you are serious about getting better **YOU MUST KEEP STRICTLY TO THE RECOMMENDATIONS!**

A very dear friend of mine had quite severe heart problems and decided to toe the line and go on a detox diet and avoid his allergens/sensitivities. In a very short space of time he was feeling better, and I had mentioned a couple of occasions the problems if you do not toe the line. Several months later he and his wife went down to Sidmouth for a walk and Bert decided to have a strawberry cream tea, as mentioned before strawberries contain high histamine, this puts stress on the adrenal glands and the cream tea exacerbated that problem, a few hours later his next door neighbour knocked on my door in a very agitated state, "come quickly I think Bert has had a stroke". I shot round the corner and up to the bedroom where he lay and it was obvious that it was more than a stroke he was dead and already cyanosed. Para medics tried to revive him but sadly he was gone.

Another patient of mine who had heart problems was fine for many months and kept strictly to the elimination of his sensitivities. He was a wealthy man and had been to Germany to buy his daughters two Hanoverian horses. On his return to the West Country he was told that the eldest daughter's boy friend, who was a chef, was preparing the evening meal. When the meal was served the starter was cream of mushroom soup! The main course was a lasagne, and he had seconds, and the sweet course was a pavlova. Hardly the meal for someone who was totally dairy free. But, and I understood when told the sequence of events, how could he be rude to the poor chef and risk upsetting the chef and his daughter, however, in hindsight he would have been better to absent himself from the meal. Several hours later he and his wife went upstairs to go to bed, he went in to the bathroom first, his wife in to the bedroom, she heard a loud crash coming from the bathroom rushed in and found him dead!

Be warned please, yes you can improve your heart condition immeasurably but on strict terms that **must**, and I repeat **must** be adhered to. I beg of you do not start on the procedure unless you are 150% committed, if you play Russian Roulette one day the bullet will get you.

Chapter 22

Kidney Conditions

Probably the most common condition I had to deal with was kidney stones, and my goodness how painful they seemed to be. I remember one man sitting on the couch being tested and perspiration pouring from him and in incredible pain. I am delighted to say that within a short space of time he was in much less pain and within months had got rid of them completely.

It probably goes without saying that if you have read this far, you will be more than aware that prevention is better than cure in every case. **Find the cause!** It is brought about by a pancreatic malfunction creating a sensitivity to certain foods and creating the oxalic calculi (stones). Which are the most common causes that I found consistently?

Milk. Butter. Cheese. Tomato. Rhubarb. Gooseberry. Strawberry. Beetroot. Spinach. Peppers. Radish.

Eliminate these for at least three months along with completing the kidney cleanse. Ring Self Health Enterprises 01342 336900. Do not be surprised if someone answers in German just say Hello and they will talk to you in English immediately. You will be recommended to take the kidney supplements for at least six weeks, and if you keep to the dietary restrictions for the 3 months recommended then you should be able to re-introduce some of the forbidden foods on a limited basis. But not dairy foods.

WHY WAIT UNTIL YOU NEED DIALYSIS OR A TRANSPLANT DO SOMETHING ABOUT IT NOW!

Kidney Cleanse

It takes a lot of liquid to "wash" the inside of your body. Taking it in the form of herbal teas gives you extra benefits. And extra enjoyment if you learn to make them with variations especial1y if you need to produce a gallon of urine a day!

Any oedema or "water holding", whether in lungs, arms, or abdomen, also requires strengthening of kidneys with this recipe. You will need:

1/2 cup dried hydrangea root *(Hydrangea arborescens)*
1/2 cup gravel root *(Eupatorium Purpureum)*
1/2 cup marshmallow root *[Aithea officinal/is)*
Black Cherry Concentrate 8 oz
Pinch vitamin B2 powder
4 bunches of fresh parsley (obtained at supermarket)
Goldenrod tincture (leave out of the recipe if you *are* allergic to it)
Ginger
Uva Ursi
Vitamin B6, 250 mg
Magnesium oxide, 300 mg
HCl drops .
Sweetening (optional)

Measure ¼ cup of each root and set them to soak, together in I 0 cups of cold tap water, using a non metal container and a non-metal lid (a dinner plate will do). Add vitamin B2 powder. After four hours (or overnight), heat to boiling and simmer *for* 20 minutes. Add black cherty concentrate and bring back to boiling. Pour through a bamboo or plastic strainer into glass jars; Drink ¼ cup by Sipping slowly throughout the day (stir in two drops HCI first). Refrigerate half to use this week, and freeze the other half for next week.

Other versions of this recipe allowed re-boiling the roots when you have finished your first batch. You need to do the kidney cleanse for six weeks to get good results, longer for severe problems.

Find fresh parsley at a grocery store. Soak it in HC1-water (1 drop per cup) with a pinch of vitamin B2 in it for 2 minutes. Drain. Cover with water and boil for I minute. Drain into glass jars. When cool enough, pour yourself half cup. Add 2 drops HCI. Sip Slowly or add to your root potion. Refrigerate a pint and freeze 1 pint. Throw away the parsley. Always add HCI at point of consuming even after pre-sterilizing.

Dose: each morning, pour together 3/4 of the root mixture and 1/2 cup parsley water, filling a large mug. Add 20 drops of goldenrod tincture and any spice, such as nutmeg, Cinnamon, etc. Then add a pinch of B2 and 4 drops HC1 to sterilize. Drink this mixture in divided doses throughout the day. Keep it cold.

Do not drink it all at once or you will get a stomach ache and feel pressure in your bladder. If your stomach is very sensitive, start on half this dose.

Also take:

Ginger capsules: one with each meal (3/day).

Uva Ursi. (one capsule worth) in the morning, and (two capsules worth) in the evening.

Vitamin B6 (250 mg): one a day.

Magnesium oxide (300 mg): one a day.

Take these supplements just before your meal to avoid burping. You do not need to duplicate the B6 and magnesium doses *if* you are already on them.

Some notes on this recipe: this herbal tea, as well as the parsley, can easily spoil. Reheat to boiling every third day if it is being stored in the refrigerator. Add HC1 drops just before

drinking. If you sterilize it in the morning you may take it to work without refrigerating it (use a glass container).

I must stress here that whilst the cleanse and removing stones is essential unless you **FIND THE CAUSE within a short space**

of time you will pollute the system again very quickly!!

Kidney Stone recipe

1/4 cup dried Hydrangea root
1/4 cup Gravel root
1/4 cup Marshmallow root
I large bunch of fresh parsley
Goldenrod tincture (leave this out of the recipe if you are allergic to it)
Ginger capsules
Uva Ursi capsules
Vegetable glycerine
Black Cherry Concentrate
Vitamin B6, 250 mg
Magnesium oxide tablets, 300 mg

Measure and set the roots to soak, together in 10 cups of cold tap water, using a non-metal container and a non-metal lid (a dinner plate will do). After four hours (or overnight) heat to boiling and simmer for 20 minutes. Drink ¼ cup as soon as it is cool enough. Pour the rest through a bamboo strainer into a sterile pint jar (glass) and several freezable containers. Refrigerate the glass jar.

Boil the fresh parsley, after rinsing, in 1 quart of water for 3 minutes. Drink ¼ cup when cool enough. Refrigerate a pint and freeze 1 pint. Throw away the parsley.

Dose: each morning, pour together 3/4 cup of the root mixture and 1/2 cup parsley water, filling a large mug. Add 2 tbs. black cherry concentrate and 20 drops of goldenrod tincture and I tbs of glycerin. Drink this mixture in divided doses throughout the day. Keep cold. Do not drink it all at once or you will get a stomach ache and feel pressure in your bladder. If your stomach is very sensitive, or you know you have kidney stones, or are over 70, start on half this dose.

Save the roots after the first boiling, storing them in the

freezer. When your supply runs low, boil them a second time, but add only 6 cups water and simmer only 10 minutes.

You may cook the roots a third time if you wish, but the recipe gets less potent. If your problem is severe, only cook them twice. Also take:

Ginger capsules: one with each meal ***(3/day)***
Uva Ursi capsules: one with breakfast and two with supper.
Vitamin B6 (250 mg): one a day.
Magnesium oxide (300 mg): one a day.

Take these supplements just before your meal to avoid burping.

Some notes on this recipe: this herbal tea, as well as the parsley, can easily spoil. Heat it to boiling every fourth day if it is being stored in the refrigerator; this re-sterilizes it. If you sterilize it in the morning you may take it to work without refrigerating it (use a glass container).

When you order your herbs, be careful! Herb companies are not the same! These roots should have a strong fragrance. If the ones you buy are barely fragrant, they have lost their active ingredients; switch to a different supplier. Fresh roots can be used. Do not use powder.

Hydrangea *(Hydrangea arborescens)* is a common flowering bush.

Gravel root *(Eupatorium purpureum)* is a wild flower.

Marshmallow root *(Alihea officinallis)* is mucilaginous and kills pain.

Fresh parsley can be bought at a grocery store. Parsley flakes and dried parsley herb do not work.

Golden rod herb works as well as the tincture but you may get an allergic reaction from smelling the herb. If you know you are allergic to this leave this one out of your recipe.

Ginger from the grocery store works fine; you may put it into capsules for yourself (size 0, 1 or 00).

There are probably dozens of herbs that can dissolve kidney stones. If you can only find several of those in the recipe, make the recipe anyway; it will just take longer' to get results. Remember that vitamin B6 and magnesium, taken daily, can prevent oxalate stones from forming. But only if you stop drinking tea. Tea has I5.6 mg oxalic acid per cup. A tall glass of iced tea could give you over 20 mg oxalic acid. Switch to herb teas. Cocoa and chocolate, also, have too much oxalic acid to be used as beverages.

Remember, too, that phosphate crystals are made when you eat too much phosphate. Phosphate levels are high in meats, breads, cereals, pastas, and carbonated drinks. Eat less and increase **your** milk (2%), fruits and vegetables. Drink at least 2 pints of water a day.

Taken from *Food Values* I4 ed by Pennington and Church 1985.

CLEANSE YOUR KIDNEYS AT LEAST TWICE A YEAR.

Obviously I can only recommend companies I have found to deliver the fresh fragrant herbs they are:-

Self Health Enterprises Ltd and Baldwin's numbers and addresses in useful numbers page.

You can dissolve all your kidney stones in 3 weeks, but make new ones in 3 days if you are drinking tea and cocoa and phosphated beverages. None of the beverage recipes in this chapter are conducive to stone formation.

Chapter 23

Gallstones

Cleansing the liver of gallstones has everything to do with gaining your health back. It dramatically improves digestion, which is the basis of your whole health. You can expect your allergies to disappear, too, more with each cleanse you do! Incredibly, it also eliminates shoulder, upper arm, and upper back pain. You have more energy and an increased sense of well being.

Cleaning the liver bile ducts is the most powerful procedure that you can do to improve your body's health.

But it should not be done before the parasite program, and for best results should follow the kidney cleanse and any dental work you need.

It is the job of the liver to make bile, 1 to 1 1/2 quarts in a day! The liver is full of tubes *(biliary tubing)* that deliver the bile to one large tube (the *common bile duct).* The gallbladder is attached to the common bile duct and acts as a storage reservoir. Eating fat or protein triggers the gallbladder to squeeze itself empty after about twenty minutes, and the stored bile finishes its trip down the common bile duct to the intestine. There are other substances that can trigger the gallbladder, such as red pepper (cayenne), ginger, and fruit acids. Note fruit juice is the first thing you have after the cleanse.

For many persons including children, the biliary tubing is choked with gallstones. Some develop allergies or hives but some have no symptoms. When the gallbladder is scanned or X-rayed nothing is seen. Typically, they are not in the gallbladder. Not only that, most are too small and not calcified, a prerequisite for visibility on X-ray. There are over *half a* dozen varieties of gallstones, most of which have cholesterol crystals in them. They can be black, red, white, green or tan coloured. The green ones get their colour from being coated with bile. At the very centre of each stone is found a clump of bacteria, suggesting a dead bit of parasite might have started the stone forming. (Author's note. Caused by a pancreatic malfunction and certain food sensitivities instigating the oxalic calculi).

As the stones grow and become more numerous the back pressure on the liver causes it to make less bile. Imagine the situation if your garden hose had marbles in it. Much less water would flow, which in turn would decrease the ability of the hose to squirt out the marbles, With gallstones, much less cholesterol leaves the. body, and cholesterol levels may rise

Gallstones, being porous, can pick up all the bacteria, *cysts,* viruses and parasites that are passing through the liver. In this way "nests" of infection are formed, forever supplying the body with fresh bacteria. No stomach infection such as ulcers or intestinal bloating can be cured permanently without removing these gallstones from the liver.

Cleanse your liver twice a year. The liver cleanse procedure as mentioned on page 88 but remember you carry out the Herbal Parasite Programme **FIRST.**

Chapter 24

Diabetes

Insulin dependent diabetes develops when the body's immune system destroys pancreatic cells that make insulin. The theory being that certain proteins in milk could stimulate the child's immune system to react adversely to proteins in pancreatic cells, which they resemble.

According to new research people with diabetes do have immune cells that seem primed to attack a cow's milk protein called beta casein which resembles the pancreatic beta cell protein. The current thinking is that this only applies to people who have a genetic disposition to the disease.

My comment has to be that every diabetic that I tested over thirty years had a pancreatic malfunction due to a sensitivity/allergen to dairy products not just milk. Of course every patient is different and there is often more than one contributory factor.

If you are a diabetic I would advise you to find a Clinical Ecologist and be tested. If that does not lower your dependency then I would definitely advise you to purchase a book called Dr Neal Barnard's Program for Reversing Diabetes (The scientifically proven system for reversing diabetes without drugs.) ISBN 978-1-50486-810-8. It is beyond doubt the most informative and advisory book about diabetes I have ever read.

Go on to the low carbohydrate Diet for Elimination of Toxins and avoid all dairy products before taking any major steps. The most important thing of all is that once again it is proof, if proof were ever needed that the pancreas is the most important organ in the body**. FIND THE CAUSE!**

A quote from the magazine Good Medicine "Just two weeks

before Dr Barnard's PBS Tour, a Government report surfaced about the dangers of Avandia, a common diabetes drug. The report found that in just 3 months in 2009, more than 300 deaths were linked to the oral medication. Dr Barnard explained to PBS viewers that a vegan diet can effectively treat diabetes and has only positive side effects". I do not think I need to make a further comment except that those figures are totally unacceptable.

Chapter 25

Cystic Fibrosis – Anorexia/Bulimia

What an incredibly distressing disease this is. I cannot say that I have treated hundreds of cases with this condition but, there have been quite a few, and the more I treated the condition the more I became convinced that the basic, and I stress the basic cause of the pancreatic malfunction was our old friend dairy products. Needless to say there were many occasions when other substances were at fault but the difference eliminating all dairy products made such a huge difference.

If you suffer from this condition then contact a Clinical Ecologist and be tested. If not applicable then by eliminating dairy you will I promise you see an enormous improvement. Mucus production is halved almost overnight. Start with the elimination of toxins diet for five days. When talking about this condition I am reminded how often I have heard opera singers like Catherine Jenkins mention the fact that they avoid dairy because it is mucus forming, and that is something you need to avoid at all costs.

ANOREXIA/BULIMIA

No book of this nature would be complete without referring to these two conditions. They are like the above very distressing conditions and most difficult for other people to understand. Having dealt with quite a number of these patients I can say without fear of contradiction that it is a pancreatic malfunction. Also beyond doubt is the origin and we are once again back to good old milk and related products. Do please exclude these and start the elimination of toxins diet for three weeks and observe, if by then you are not seeing a dramatic change then consult a

Clinical Ecologist as soon as possible. It is also interesting to note that milk and dairy products in general have been scientifically proven to be related to self harming.

If you are interested enough to pick this book up, like many, you may well rifle through the pages to see if there is anything that suits you. Therefore I have put as an Appendix A, information that you need to know even before you begin to go to the chapter that interests you.

THINGS YOU NEED TO KNOW

Real salt

Common table salt is a heavily refined substance containing only sodium chloride plus additives. The refining process includes washing or boiling the salt, adding strong chemicals and exposing the salt to extreme heat. It is then mixed with iodine, bleaching and anti- caking agents to create the bright white free-flowing product sold in shops. Because nearly everyone uses table salt, this is the salt used in medical research which, correctly, has found it to be damaging to health.

Most commercial sea salts are also refined' in the sense that the way in which they are harvested loses nearly all of their minerals and trace elements (called bitterns).

Unrefined sea salt

Because every attempt to keep the bitterns is made, unrefined sea salts (like 'Celtic Sea Salt') contain all 84 trace elements and micronutrient found in the sea. it can both lower high blood pressure and raise low blood pressure, and help rehydrate cells by removing extracellular fluid.

Interestingly, the large amount of extracellular fluid in the human body (typically three gallons in an adult) is a powerful argument that we evolved in the sea. The mineral content and balance of the two are almost identical. Diluted sea water is used as a tonic and has been found to reduce the sticking of blood platelets to cell walls.

Magnesium The major mineral in unrefined sea salt is. magnesium, adequate levels of which are essential to good health. Magnesium salts, for instance, stimulate white blood cell activity in the immune system, enhance the action of vitamins and enzymes, help process glucose and phosphocalcium, and help rid the body of any excess sodium. Magnesium deficiency is a significant contributory factor in many diseases. It can be caused by consuming grains, vegetables and fruit grown on chemically fertilised or pesticide sprayed fields, by consuming white bread and refined grain products (refining whole wheat and polishing rice can remove 80% of their magnesium), and by using refined salt. Refined table salt contains either no or less than OO3% magnesium salts, and commercial sea salts contain usually around 0.1%, instead of the 4%-1% average content in unrefined sea salt.

Sodium. Adequate supplies of sodium are also essential, as sodium combines with water and various ions (e.g. chlorine, potassium, calcium, hydrogen) to help many body functions. Sodium chloride, for instance, plays an important part in the primary process of digestion and absorption by activating the primary enzyme in the mouth, salivary amylase. In the parietal cells of the stomach wall, it is used to make hydrochloric acid, essential to good digestion. Inadequate levels of sodium chloride can:

- raise blood pressure
- accelerate ageing
- cause liver failure, kidney problems, and massive adrenal exhaustion
- tire the heart muscles, increasing the risk of heart attack

Blood Pressure

A Dutch study (covering 100 men and women aged 55-75 years

of age with mild to moderately high blood pressure) found that, when table salt (98% sodium chloride) was replaced with an unrefined salt high in magnesium and potassium, reductions in blood pressure equivalent to that obtained with blood pressure-reducing drugs was achieved.' A reduction in pulse rate was also recorded. in the group given the unrefined salt. The benefits fell off after the study, suggesting that unrefined, mineral-rich salt needs to be a permanent part of the diet.

Low blood pressure is also unhealthy, causing, for example, low energy, cold hands and feet, dry skin and poor memory. Unrefined sea salt can also raise low blood pressure. For more information on Celtic Sea Salt and Sea Water Therapy ring Regenerative Nutrition on 01892 512337.

Beware of Calpol

Calpol, like many medicines, is simply a symptom suppressant. It has become part of western culture, administered unquestioningly to the youngest babies at the slightest suggestion of discomfort or infection. Every symptom is caused by a beneficial, intelligent immune system response to something not quite right in the body. They should never be suppressed unless the child is obviously in severe pain and a diagnosis has been made.

There are other good reasons for not resorting to Calpol – in particular, its ingredients:

- Paracetamol, potentially fatal when used too regularly or above the recommended dose. Never administer Calpol without consulting a doctor if the child has kidney or liver problems
- Carmoisine (strawberry flavour E122), associated with hyperactivity, asthma, hives and insomnia
- Glycerol (E422), can cause headaches, thirst, nausea and high blood sugar
- Sorbitol (E420), associated with flatulence, diarrhoea and

bloating
- Methyl hydroxybenzoate (E218), can cause hyperactivity, asthma, skin problems, insomnia and numb mouth
- Xanthan gum (E415), can cause asthma, skin irritation and hay fever

Once the source of discomfort or pain has been identified, there are homoeopathic remedies which can he administered in complete safety even every 5-10 minutes to soothe symptoms. Aconite, a general remedy always worth trying first, is good at nipping colds, fevers and inflammation in the bud if administered quickly enough. Belladonna is best for high fever, Chamomillais good for teething pains, as is Pulsatilla for ear infections. If meningitis is suspected, ring **999** immediately and alternate Aconite and Belladonna every five minutes.

Always call a doctor if:

- a fever is accompanied by vomiting
- a fever lasts longer than 48 hours
- the Child becomes sensitive to light or develops a stiff neck
- there is a skin rash (especially one that does not whiten when pressed)
- the child's temperature is over I O5 Fahrenheit
- the child is less than four months old
- the child makes prolonged, high pitch screams
- a head injury is followed by vomiting and/or fever

For further information visit Tracey's website:

www.roadbacktohealth.co.uk

Ed. (i) We recommend you register with a local homoeopath who can advice you on first aid remedies to have at home and whom you can consult when your child is sick.

(ii) Unsuspected by most parents, many baby medicines

contain paracetamol. Even parents aware of the dangers find it extremely difficult to ensure that maximum limits are not exceeded when combining medicines.

(iii) Paracetamol *is* one of the commonest causes of liver failure in the UK. If it were submitted for licensing today it would not gain the approval of the UK's Committee on Safety of Medicines as an over the-counter drug. It has been associated with kidney damage and asthma. (iv) Some researchers caution against using drugs to block *fever* in case it interferes with normal immune development in the brain, resulting in neurological disorders in susceptible children.

(11104) TraceyDennIs. Intormed Parent *15.O4pi3*

BULLET POINTS

Whenever possible BUY ORGANIC

1. Use a non-fluoride toothpaste (Health shop)
2. Avoid deodorants that contain aluminium (health shop)
3. Make sure you use natural feminine hygiene products (Health shop)
4. Use organic cotton buds, cotton wool
5. Use colloidal silver sticking plasters
6. Use non biological and natural washing products. Essential for babies bedding and clothing.
7. Use non toxic paints without solvents
8. Avoid cooking in tap water and drinking tap water
9. Avoid water in soft plastic water bottles and never leave in cars to get warm
10. If you are advised to have an X-Ray then ring Galen Pharmacy 01305 26399 and order homoeopathic X-Ray 30. Take a dose of once daily morning and night for 3 days
11 Scans? Take Radium 30 from above source, including ultra sound pregnancy scans
12. To combat the effects of vaccination take Thuja 30 for five days morning and night. Also ring Self Health Enterprises

01342 336900 and ask for CELA 2M.

13. Wasp stings homoeopathic Vespa Vulgaris 30 and place under tongue every 15 minutes until all swelling disappears. Bee stings – Apis Mellifica 30 and use same procedure.
14. Hay fever – Sinapis Nigra 30 and take every 15 minutes until symptoms disappear then once daily during season.
15. For those affected in swimming baths take Chlorinum 30 half an hour before swimming and after swimming is completed.
16. Avoid air fresheners other than essential oils.
17. Use as many natural cleaning products such as lemon juice, bicarbonate of soda, vinegar etc as seen on TV.
18. Use whole-foods and beverages instead of processed and packaged foods and-synthetic canned drinks wherever possible.
19. Sunshine contrary to what you are told is vital for health Vitamin D3. DO NOT use sun blocks only natural oils. Regular exercise and fresh air are also vital.
20. All of these will be useful but the most useful of all is a HEALTHY ORGANICDIET.

Diet Sheet For Elimination of Toxins/Migraine and Gut Migraine

ON RISING

Glass of hot water with teaspoon of honey.

BREAKFAST

Corn flakes, shredded wheat, puffed rice, goat, sheep or organic soya milk. Fruit juice of choice (non citric), Darjeeling, Assam, Luaka or Green tea, Caro, Barley cup, Pionier (alternative coffee).

LUNCH

Salad – organic whenever possible. Lettuce, cress, cucumber, celery, grated or shredded cabbage, beetroot, vegetarian cheese, one ryvita or slice of wheatmeal bread, beef, lamb, chicken, top fish only.(NO BOTTOM FISH plaice, dab, flounder etc;).

TEA

Wheatmeal bread and honey, tea or alternative coffee.

SUPPER

Avocado, Icelandic prawns, steak, lamb chops, chicken, cod, whiting, haddock, Pollock, bream, bass. Boiled or baked potato (no skin), peas, beans, lentils, cabbage, sprouts, broccoli, cauliflower, carrots.

Producing alkaline but acid in raw state

Grapefruit, orange, lemon, limes.

Alkaline in raw state but acid when cooked

Beef, lamb, chicken, pork.

Foods which can cause constipation

Coffee, cheese, salt meat, white bread, spiced foods, mixed dishes, eggs, rice, pastry, soya, condiments, pickles, tea.

Foods which can have a laxative effect

Raisins, raw cabbage, apples, whole-wheat, figs, plums, prunes, pears, tomato, cauliflower, peaches, grapes, celery, grapefruit, bran, spinach, parsnips, swede, carrots.

As constipation is the scourge of society today it is worth bearing these foods in mind. This diet plan and the foods suggested are advisory and for you to chose from. Please remember the importance of drinking enough water on a daily basis. 3 litres is minimum recommended.

You will note that I have eliminated Citrus/Bioflavinoids for migraine patients.

DO NOT drink with a meal. The salivary glands produce

ample water to aid mastication:

drinking fluid with a meal impairs and enfeebles these glands.

NO PORK, HAM, BACON, VEAL. APPLE SKIN. APPLE JUICE. CIDER, CIDER VINEGAR.

ASPALLS OR PEAKES ORGANIC APPLE JUICE IS PERMITTED.

THIS DIET IS FOR FIVE DAYS AS A DETOX DIET – IT IS THEN LEFT TO YOUR

COMMON SENSE TO EXPAND YOUR DIET WITH CAUTION.

Water

"The great bulk of evidence from numerous studies therefore supports a link between aluminium consumption, especially monomeric aluminium from drinking water, and an elevated incidence of Alzheimer's disease. Harold D. Foster, PHd.2005".

This is a subject that needs to follow on from fluoridation and some comments need to be made about chlorination. I am not trying to scare the pants off you, I just wish to make it clear that there are hazards. There is a minefield out there and you must learn to cross it safely. Hopefully, with me "holding your hand", we can cross it safely together and lead a healthier life. Chlorine certainly kills germs - but what else does it kill? When water is drawn from lakes and rivers rather than underground surface, it comes into contact with soil, silt, mud and effluent. This interaction produces compounds called trihalomethanes (THMs) the most well known being chloroform. Chloroform is a known carcinogen, causing gastrointestinal and urinary tract cancers. Chlorine itself has been linked to high blood pressure, anaemia, arthritis and diabetes and is a contributor to heart disease. Even in a minute quantity sufficient to kill germs, chlorine can undermine the body's defences against artheroscierosis — the hardening and thickening of the arteries.WDDTY,Vo13.No12.

If a plant in your garden fails to grow properly, you may add nutrients to the soil and you will certainly add water. If the water is contaminated you know the plant will be affected. What makes you think this has no bearing on your own health? Clean water is essential to our health. Let's face it we are 80% water. It affects our cells, our enzymatic processes and our ability to detoxify.

Is it possible to name one particular ingredient that is harmful? I don't think so, but it is not difficult to imagine that a cocktail of chemicals could be lethal. The Swedes still blame us for the industrial revolution that precipitated the clouds of acid rain which destroyed fish stocks in their lakes. Falling rain deposits, smoke, dust, chemical fumes, germs, lead and strontium 90 fell on the land. . Rain water then flowed through the soil, flowed into rivers and streams picking up fertilisers and pesticides, as well as herbicides, nitrates and nitrites. We are once again committed to thinking about our cars, and whether we would chose to put the wrong fuel in and expect to get a good performance. Water is so basic to our health that we need to give it very serious consideration.

The simplest and best method to remove contamination is to use a reverse osmosis filter. Having investigated and used various methods of water purification it is reverse osmosis that proved the most satisfactory for me. The back up service is also second to none and the company I use is On Tap Water Supplies, based in Somerton, Somerset. Telephone no 01458274289.

It is not the cheapest method by any means, but to my knowledge it is certainly the most effective as can be seen from the following: The most common impurities measured in parts per million (PPM). I would advise using a multi-mineral supplement to offset any lack of minerals in RO water.

Tap water 400-700 ppm

Jug filtered tap water 275 ppm

Plastic bottled mineral water 175 ppm

Reverse osmosis 6 ppm

So, as you can see a vast difference and I would suggest economical common sense.

In his book *Your Body's Many Cries For Water,* Dr Batmanghelidj recommends that you drink at least two litres of water a day. He also states that dehydration can be responsible for a huge range of ailments and degenerative disease. In the UK now we use sodium fluoride not calcium fluoride for adding fluorine to water. Sodium fluoride is banned in the countries previously mentioned. It was used originally as a rat poison and is a by-product of the aluminium industry.

A detailed review paper published in March 2002 discussed powerful evidence that aluminium from drinking water and other sources was a major contributory factor to Alzheimer's disease.

It was thought for many years that it was impossible for substances to cross the blood/brain barrier. Research now shows that aluminium can react with fluoride in water, and this causes more aluminium to cross the blood brain barrier and deposit in the brain. If there are old pipes in the house then these ought to be renewed, as chemicals deposited from streams can lead to lead, copper and mercury contamination.

So, what is the answer to combat these problems? Bottled and spring water is not the complete answer, as storage in plastic containers for any length of time leads to contamination by synthetic estrogens.

Carbon jug filters are good for reducing chlorine content but not good at leaching out many other contaminants. They also need changing quite frequently.

Ceramic filters are quite expensive but they do remove heavy metals, nitrates, fluoride and bacteria. The weakness is that there is poor removal of organic compounds like pesticides, dioxins and estrogens.

Distilled water. Distillation plants are expensive but they do produce the purest water. It has been suggested that it leaches minerals from the body and the bone structure. I do not think this can be true as thousands of kidney patients using distilled water in dialysis machines show no loss of mineral content in their bodies. Reverse Osmosis. What are the advantages? It is plumbed in with state of the art carbon technology. It uses a membrane under pressure to separate relatively pure water or other solvents from a less pure solution.

Potentially Harmful Ingredients Used in the Personal Care Industry

This is as good a time as any to bring to your attention some of the potentially harmful ingredients commonly used by the personal care industry:

Alcohol

A colourless, volatile, inflammable liquid produced by the fermentation of yeast and carbohydrates. Alcohol is used frequently as a solvent and is also found in beverages and medicine. As an ingredient in ingestible products, alcohol may cause body tissues to be more vulnerable to carcinogens. Mouthwashes with an alcohol content of 25% or more have been implicated in mouth and tongue cancers. This is obviously implicated in candida albicans, and in most cases there is pre-disposition to this complaint, causing an imbalance in gut flora.

Elastin of High Molecular Weight

A protein similar to collagen that is the main component of elastic fibres. Elastin is also derived from animal sources. Its effect on the skin is similar to collagen.

Fluorocarbons

A colourless, non-flammable gas or liquid that can produce mild upper respiratory tract irritation. Fluorocarbons are commonly used as a propellant in hair sprays.

Formaldehyde

A toxic, colourless gas that is an irritant and a carcinogen. When combined with water, formaldehyde is used as a disinfectant, fixative or preservative. Formaldehyde is found in many cosmetic products and conventional nail care systems.

Petrolatum

A petroleum based grease that is used industrially as a grease component. Petrolatum exhibits many of the same potentially harmful properties as mineral oil.

Propylene Glycol

A cosmetic form of mineral oil found in automatic brake and hydraulic fluid and industrial anti-freeze. In skin and hair products, propylene glycol works as a humescent, which is a substance that retains the moisture content of skin or cosmetic products by preventing the escape of moisture or water. Material Safety Data Sheets (MSD'S) warn users to avoid skin contact with propylene glycol as this strong skin irritant can cause liver abnormalities and kidney damage.

Alpha Hydroxy Acid

An organic acid produced by anaerobic respiration. Skin care products containing AHA exfoliate not only damage skin cells but the skins protective barrier as well. Long-term skin damage may result from its use.

Glycerin

A syrupy liquid that is chemically produced by combining water and fat. Glycerin is used as a solvent and a plasticiser. Unless the humidity of air is over 65%, glycerin draws moisture from the lower layer of the skin and holds it on the surface, which dries the skin from the inside out.

Kaolin

A fine white clay used in making porcelain. Like bentonite, kaolin smothers and weakens the skin.

SodiumLauryl Sulphate(SLS)

An anionic surfacant used in cosmetics and industrial chemicals as a cleansing agent. Used as a thickener and a foaming agent in shampoos, toothpastes, and cleansers, and as a wetting agent in garage floor cleaners, engine degreasers, and auto cleaning products. SLS is used around the world in clinical studies as a skin irritant. High levels of skin penetration may occur at even low concentrations. Studies have shown SLS to have a degenerate effect on the cell membrane due to its protein denaturing properties. It can also maintain residual levels in major organs of the body from skin contact. Carcinogenic nitrates can form in the manufacturing of SLS or by its combination with other nitrogen bearing ingredients within a formulation, creating a nitrosating agent.

Aluminium

A metallic element used extensively in the manufacture of aircraft components, prosthetic devices and as an ingredient in antiperspirants, antacids and antiseptics. Aluminium has been linked to Alzheimer's disease.

Animal Fat (Tallow)

A type of animal tissue made up of oily solids or semisolids that are water insoluble esters of glycerol with fatty acids.

Animal fats and lye are the chief ingredients in a bar of soap; a cleaning and emulsifying product that may act as a breeding ground for bacteria.

Lanolin

A fatty substance extracted from wool which is frequently found in cosmetics and lotions. Lanolin is a common skin sensitiser that can cause allergic reactions, such as skin rashes.

Lye

A highly concentrated watery solution of sodium hydroxide or potassium hydroxide. Lye is combined with animal fats to make bars of soap, which may corrode and dry out the skin.

SodiumLaureth Sulphate (SLES)

SLES is the alcohol form (ethoxylated) of SLS. It has higher foaming qualities and is slightly less irritating, but may cause more drying. May also cause potentially carcinogenic formulation of nitrates, or nitrosating agents, by reacting with other ingredients.

Bentonite

A porous clay that expands to many times its dry volume as it absorbs water. Bentonite, commonly found in many cosmetic foundations, may clog pores and suffocate skin.

Collagen

An insoluble fibrous protein that is too large to penetrate the skin. This collagen, found in most skin care products, is derived from animal skins and ground up chicken feet. This ingredient forms a layer of film that may suffocate the skin.

Mineral oil

A derivative of crude oil (petroleum) that is used industrially as a cutting fluid and lubricating oil. Mineral oil forms an oily film over the skin to lock in any moisture, toxins and wastes, but hinders normal skin respiration by keeping oxygen out.

Talc

A soft grey-green powder used in some personal hygiene and

cosmetic products, inhaling talc may be harmful as this substance is recognised as a potential carcinogen.

Dioxins

A potentially carcinogenic by product that results from the process used to bleach paper at paper mills. Dioxin treated containers sometimes transfer dioxins to the product itself.

Journal of the American College of Toxicology. Volume 2.

This information is not designed to alarm you, but to make you aware that not everything is quite what it seems. Not only in the food industry but in every industry. For instance in tea bags and more importantly where women are concerned it is used to bleach tampons and sanitary towels. Go to your health shop and get the natural varieties. Also think about obtaining alternative healthy soaps.

What are the nutrient destroyers? See also Chapter 10 – Candida Albicans

- Aspirin destroys - Vit **A-** calcium – potassium – **B** Complex – Vit C.
- Caffeine destroys - B1- inositol – biotin – potassium – zinc.
- Chlorine destroys Vit E.
- Chocolate contains caffeine and fat.
- Fluoride destroys - Vit C.
- Sedatives destroy folic acid - Vit D.
- Menstruation -iron -B12 - calcium -magnesium.
- Stress destroys all vitamin/mineral stores.
- White sugar and flour - B complex.

Antibiotics prescribed and also added to animal feed destroy vitamin stores and create an imbalance. This in turn creates a continual battle for the immune system to remain stable.

When you take antibiotics you not only kill the bad bacteria but the good as well. It is rare that you will hear a physician discussing the fact that one side of antibiotic therapy is the disruption of good intestinal bacteria. Be assured that when healthy bacteria are destroyed there is **always** a price to pay! How many times have I heard lady patients telling me that when they took a course of antibiotics they suffered with thrush.

Antibiotics

When penicillin was discovered it was thought we had a magic bullet. It would kill all bacteria and cure all bacterial infections. Life would be so wonderful if it was as simple as that. Pop a pill and all will be well. Of course it did not work like that and unfortunately we have had the hard lesson to learn, that by using antibiotics as the cure-all, the bullet has turned on us and shot us in the foot. Bacteria learn to adapt and become resistant, our former wonder drugs are now all but useless. Did you realise that antibiotics only treat bacteria. Many of the deadly infections today are caused by viruses and antibiotics are useless against them. We can be infected by fungi too, and antibiotics encourage fungal growth. Consider this point carefully please: - Every time you take an antibiotic you are giving the bacteria around you a new opportunity to develop resistance. Remember my comments about organic food - every time you eat milk, cheese, eggs and most meats, unless they are organic, you are being exposed to antibiotics. Livestock are given daily doses virtually from birth, because antibiotics are growth promoters, and keep milk and eggs fresh for much longer, thus increasing farmer's profits.

So, what is the consequence? Fewer and fewer antibiotics are effective against deadly infections. Patients who contract serious infections like pneumonia, or pick up a hospital infection like the deadly staphylococcus, often die because the bacteria are so resistant. The recent E-Coli outbreak in Scotland is a typical example. In America, New York in particular, tuberculosis is becoming epidemic, it is quoted as affecting as many as 1 in 3 of the population, and it is antibiotic resistant. Do not be complacent it is also making a comeback in the United Kingdom too.

Because of antibiotic abuse we have lost the 'war'. Remember the last major outbreak of Influenza in this country. It was in the winter of 1996/7 and thousands of people were affected. It lingered on for months and what were many told when they went to their GP, "well, you have influenza but there is nothing I can do for you or give you as they do not work, so go home and it will burn itself out eventually". I do not wish to sound anti GP because if there were to be a secondary infection, or a suspicion of it, then antibiotics would be prescribed. But it really does not inspire confidence when it is publicly stated that antibiotics are not effective in these viral conditions. Think long and hard please, there are alternative ways of approaching illness of any kind; protecting and strengthening the immune system is one way of doing just that. What happens when we get a scare that chicken flu (never happened) or swine flu (never happened), we are told there are vaccines available, and what are the ingredients of these vaccines? Who makes the money? The pharmaceutical companies in every single case. If they are not used in this country as with Tamiflu then they are shipped to countries such as Africa.

Alexander Fleming, who discovered penicillin warned nearly a century ago that overuse of antibiotics would create resistant bacteria.

Pesticides, Sprays

If you know anything about modern food production you will not need me to tell you that pesticides and sprays are in constant use. I referred earlier to the pesticides and sprays being used on pastureland, nitrites, nitrates, growth promoters, weed killers etc. The cattle feed on this and it ends up in our meat and milk. Weed killers are used to spray the potato crop while growing and again when they are put down for storage and now of course GM Foods being used in cattle feed..

When my wife was asked, several years or so ago, and as a favour for a friend of ours, to collect the pesticides for his potato crop she had to sign three poison forms. A patient of mine is a very large potato grower in Kent, and when I mentioned about not eating the potato skins when baked, the reply I received was, "don't be silly, we would not eat those, we have a large patch for our own consumption".

Buy ORGANIC!! Your apples are sprayed so often it is unbelievable, and I have yet to test a patient who does not react to apple skin. Buy ORGANIC!! If they are not organic then please make sure you peel them. I am beginning to sound like a one-man advertising campaign for the Soil Association. They do an admirable job and you will see the Soil Association logo on foods that are acceptably organic. But that is not the reason I am mentioning these things, I am referring to clinical reactions, not just test results, but also the reports I receive from patients who have ingested something unsuitable. These reactions can be quite severe and often take as long as five days to clear the system and as long as three weeks for balanced health to return. So beware!! I would like to quote from a book called 'The Pesticide Conspiracy' by Professor Robert Van Den Bosch, it is the last page, *"Nature is emitting signals warning us that under the existing format the future is ominous. She is saying that we cannot continue our attempts to ruthlessly dominate her and that if we persist disaster is in the offing. She has many voices, and of the clearest is that of the insects. The insects have already told us that we cannot overwhelm them and that there has been a price to pay in trying.*

But, Nature has other voices and, if we listen carefully, we can hear these additional warnings too: the voices of the trees in the crashing forests before an assault of axes, the later rumble of a mudslide as a cloudburst sweeps the denuded mountainside, the voice of the soil in the crunch of the alkali beneath the boots of a farmer pacing his land ruined by bad irrigation; the voice of the water as it roars crystal clear through the pen stocks of a mighty dam, leaving behind the nutrients that once nourished a great floodplain and fed a vast fishery; the voice of the wind as it hisses with a load of dust whipped from the topsoil of half a county. Yes, the voices of Nature are quite easy to hear - if we will only listen. The question is, will we? And if we do, can we overcome our corrupt ways and marshal our efforts to collaborate with Nature as her brightest child and shepherd of Earth's life system? If not, it is almost certain that things will worsen for Nature, but even more so for us. Then at a certain point in time we may no longer be able to cope with the adversity and we will perish. But Nature will survive, and so, too, will the insects, her most successful children. And as a final bit of irony, it will be the insects that polish the bones of the very last of us to fall."

This was written and published in 1978. It does not take a lot of imagination to realise how prophetic these words were .Look at the threat we are under with the extinction of so many bee colonies. For thirty two years later we are seeing the natural resources of this world threatened, and the natural kingdom occupying the land and the sea being polluted to the point of extinction. Is it really surprising that fishermen patients of mine tell me that they would never touch the fish, or let their families do so, because they are so diseased through pollution. Potato growers who will not eat the produce they sell to the public, apple growers who save private orchards for their own consumption, the list is endless. Just consider the billions of pounds spent on additives and preservatives in this country alone, and you will see why there are cartels to protect them, and intentionally deprive you of the information that is rightly yours.(Conspiracy at its worst).

It really depends on you the public demanding NATURAL foods, uncontaminated by pesticides and sprays, additives and preservatives, genetically engineered, or irradiated so that those in power will listen and act upon the pressure you exert. Even politicians realise that it is the public that put them in office, so contact your local Member of Parliament if you have a complaint.

ESSENTIAL VITAMINS AND MINERALS

Magnesite is a natural magnesium mineral which is essential for good bone structure. It is essential for the metabolism of vitamin B6 and enters into many enzyme processes in the body. The parathyroids require magnesium for the proper control of calcium in the bones. (See Shils ME. 1976 Magnesium Deficiency and Calcium and Parathyroid Interrelations P.23-46 in Trace Elements in Health and Disease Vol. 2 Prasad and Oberleas Academic Press NY).

Pyridoxine/Vitamin B6 has been used to treat rheumatism as it reduces edema, joint stiffness, pain and sensory numbness, especially in the arms. (Dr. Ellis, *The Doctor's Report* 1973).

Zinc is essential for many bodily functions, especially for the proper cross linking of connective tissue in cartilage, and for its regeneration (See Prasad and Oberleas as above).

Silica or Diatomite contains silicon which is essential for normal growth in all animals and man. Its deficiency causes depressed growth and abnormal bone formation. It is essential for mucopolysaccharide metabolism and proper cartilage formation (See Davis N.T. 1981. *An Appraisal of the Newer Trace Elements* P. 173-174 in *Trace Element Deficiency; Metabolic and Physiological Consequences.* Ed. Fowden, Garton and Mills. Royal Soc. London).

Vitamin B3 Niacin is a component of 2 co-enzymes, NAD and NADP, essential for cell respiration as well as being involved in fat and protein synthesis and is reported to help arthritic conditions. (Doctor Hoffer, *The Complete Book of Vitamins,* 1977).

Pantothenate - Vitamin B5 has been used to treat rheumatism as it aids tissue repair. Rheumatoid arthritics have low blood levels of this vitamin according to Drs Barton- Wright and Elliot *(Lancet,* October 1963).

Kelp is rich in iodine and boron; both these help to stimulate the parathyroid glands which in turn control the calcium in bones.

Devil's Claw is an African herb that has long been recognised as useful for arthritis.

Manganese is essential for many enzyme processes and in proper use of many of the B Vitamins, which in turn help arthritic conditions. Muscular rheumatism is helped by manganese. Zinc and manganese work together to control the body levels of other heavy metals. It is found mainly in whole grains and green leaf vegetables.

Copper is essential for the proper formation of haemoglobin and red blood cells. Arthritics need adequate blood to carry around the necessary minerals and other bone forming substances. Cartilage must also be repaired and blood helps here. Some elderly people tend towards anaemia so the blood must be built up in order to help them properly. Very little is needed but that small amount is necessary.

Calcium Fluoride is very sparingly soluble but it is absorbed through the intestine. When incorporated into the bones as calcium fluoroapatite it gives hardness and strength to the bone crystals. It stimulates osteoblastic activity and so helps in formation of new bone, especially after damage. Very little is needed but it certainly helps in many cases of osteoarthritis, rheumatoid arthritis, osteoporosis and ankylosing spondylitis. (See Blackmores Prescribers Reference A.8.1).

Molybdenum helps to prevent dental caries which are really poor bone growth of the teeth, so other bones are likely to be similarly affected. Together with zinc it helps to counter the effect of other heavy metals. It is found in whole grains, seeds, beans, nuts and eggs.

Selenium is an anti-oxidant and will aid in the metabolism of Vitamin E. It is essential for the proper functioning of muscles and is a must for muscular rheumatism. It is present in garlic, whole grains, meat and eggs. Men and animals cannot live without it but we only need 200 micro grams daily. Remember many arthritics cannot break down wholemeal flour.

Cobalt is part of the Vitamin B12 or hydroxycobalamin. We need very little of it but it is essential for the liver and proper blood formation. It is present in meat foods, especially liver (organic only) and vegetarians are often short of this vitamin. Its presence ensures better growth and resistance to disease. Pregnancy makes big demands on the body's reserves of this vitamin because the developing foetus must get it for proper growth.

Bee Pollen is a natural source of boron and is rich in trace elements.

Equisetum/Horse Tail is a herb rich in silica and this helps to harden bones.

Here is a list of seventeen additives which will, in time, be proven to be harmful to the human system over a period of years.

1. BUTYLATED HYDROXYANISOLE - E 320.(BHA)
2. BUTYLATED HYDROXYTOLUENE -E 321 (BHT)
3. DISODIUM DIHYDROGEN PHOSPHATASE.
4. MONOSODIUM GLUTAMATE - SODIUM HYDROGEN L-GLUTAMATE E621.
5. CARAGEENAN - E407.
6. FOOD COLOURINGS.
7. SODIUM NITRATE - E 250/25 1.
8. SODIUM NITRITE.
9. POLYSORBATE 60- E 435.
10. POLYSORBATE 80- E 433.
11. DI-POTASSIUM PHOSPHATE - E 340(b).
12. SORBITAN-MONOSTEARATE - E 491.
13. OXYGEN INTERCEPTOR.
14. SULPHUR DIOXIDE - E 220.
15. BENZOATE OF SODA - E 211.

16 SODIUM SILICO ALUMINATE.
17 CARAMEL-E 150.

Things to remember

Make sure you refrigerate oils once they are opened.

Do not re-heat oils. Use once and dispose of it.

Avoid freezing ready cooked meals then re-heating them.

Avoid re-heating meals of any kind.

Fry or roast food with oils rather than margarine. Reserve these for cakes and pastries and eat them cold.

Avoid microwaved food entirely. It alters blood platelets within 15 minutes of ingestion whether it be cooked, thawed or refrigerated.

Use Non-Fluoride toothpaste. There are also herbal toothpaste's without fluoride available in most Health Shops.

Avoid pasteurised goat or sheep milks where possible. The body does not cope easily with the altered state of the milk.

Avoid aluminium cookware if possible. Better to use stainless steel, glass, or enamel cookware.

Avoid overcooking food because carbon particles are deleterious.

Constipation

It really is quite amazing how many patients report this as a life long problem. Some actually report that it is common for them to only go once a week. I need not tell you that this is not normal and certainly will not be allowable. It is essential, as far as I am concerned, that you pass a motion at least once daily - preferably twice.

One thing I would not wish you to do is to take Senokot or any other purgative. There are various aids to help with this problem. The one that seems to suit everybody is Linusit Gold from your local health shop. Or Carrefour from Argyll Herbs, Herbilax is another. The most natural way is with magnesium ascorbate - Vitamin C. This is in capsule or powder form and is available from Biocare Ltd (Tel:0121 433 3727). This can be taken without any side effects until the stool is loose. If it turns to diarrhoea then cut back slightly. On the first day take one teaspoon in organic juice or water morning and night. If there is no motion the following morning then add a further teaspoon at lunch time and continue increasing by a teaspoon each day until relief is obtained. A teaspoon is equivalent to 4 grams so if you are taking tablets equate the dosage. You may find that, after being on the Arthritic way of eating for three weeks, the bowel settles down and no problems are encountered. Should the problem continue then consult your practitioner as there are tests that can be carried out to ascertain the problem .As a precaution drink 2 glasses of filtered water before breakfast.

Appendix A

USEFUL ADDRESSES

GREEN LIBRARY
6,RICKETT STREET
LONDON
SW6 1RU

NUTRI CENTRE
7,PARK CRESCENT
LONDON
08456026744

KIERON & ANNE McGRATH
THE BELL & BIRDTABLE
RUNNINGTON
WELLINGTON
SOMERSET
01823 663O80

BIOCARE LTD
180, LIFFORD LANE
KINGS NORTON
B IRMINGHAM
B30 3NT
0121 433 3727

HILDRETH & COCKER
DAVID ROWLANDS
01275340042 0800 3166714

SELF HEALTH ENTERPRISES LTD,
BULLRUSHES FARM ,
COOMBE HILL ROAD,
EAST GRINSTEAD,
WEST SUSSEX.
RH19 4LZ
01342 336900

ROGER SANDERS
5 FAR STREET
WYMESWOLD
LEICESTER
LE12 6TZ
01509 880447 (If difficulties send wellbeing.research@ virgin.net)

G.BALDWIN &CO HERBALISTS
171/173 WALWORTH ROAD
LONDON SE17 1RW
0207 703 5550

GOOD VITALITY LTD (CHRIS HYSLOP)
HIGHLANDS CLOSE
CRAWLEY
W.SUSSEX RH10 6RX
01293 446244
Colloidal silver. Zappers. Batteries etc.

FORESIGHT THE ASSOCIATION FOR PRE-CONCEPTUAL CARE
28, THE PADDOCK
GODALMING
SURREY
GU7 1XD
01243868001

ARGYLL HERBS DIRECT
15 DARBY ROAD
BISHOPS LYDEARD
SOMERSET
TA4 3BB
08458630679

ON TAP WATER TREATMENT
BANCOMBE TRADING ESTATE.
SOMERTON
SOMERSET
01458 274289

WDDTY
4, WALLACE ROAD
LONDON
NI 2PG
0207 354 4592

GALEN PHARMACY
LEWELL MILL
WEST STAFFORD
DORCHESTER
DORSET
01305 263996 FOR HOMOEOPATHIC PREPARATIONS.

Appendix B

CLINICAL ECOLOGISTS TRAINED BY GWYNNE H. DAVIES
D.Sc.ND.DO.FEMA.(Ret'd)

SEAN EMMERSON
20 MELROSE ROAD
NORWICH
NR4 7PN
01603 503600

KAZY VINCENT-JANES
BETCHWORTH HOUSE
CHIDEOCK
DT6 6JW
01297 489894

JUNE STAPLEY
24 LYTE LANE
WEST CHARLETON
KINGSBRIDGE
DEVON
TQ7 2BW
01548531643

PAMELA HAYHURST
154 MARLOW ROAD
PAIGNTON
DEVON
TQ3 3ND
01803552562

Index